A SURVIVAL GUIDE FOR COSMETOLOGISTS

TIPS FROM THE TRENCHES

by Karen Levine and Alan Gelb

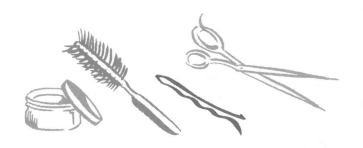

THOMSON

DELMAR LEARNI

Australia   Canad
Spain   United Kii

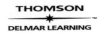

A Survival Guide for Cosmetologists
by Karen Levine & Alan Gelb

Business Unit Executive Director:
Susan L. Simpfenderfer

Developmental Editor:
Patricia Gillivan

Executive Production Manager:
Wendy A. Troeger

Cover Design:
Kristina Almquist

Executive Marketing Manager:
Donna J. Lewis

Channel Manager:
Stephen Smith

NOTICE TO THE READER

CONTENTS

Acknowledgments

The author and Delmar would like to express their gratitude to the following professionals who offered numerous, valuable suggestions:

Dianne Atchley

Letha Barnes

Kathy Earl

Patti Ferraro

Stacy Heatherly

Jane Kane

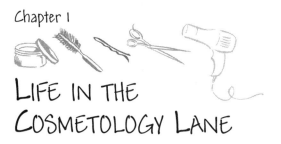

Chapter 1

LIFE IN THE COSMETOLOGY LANE

Congratulations! Here you are, working in your chosen profession, making a very respectable living, and feeling good about your accomplishments. You are in a strong and positive place. But it has taken time to get to this place and the road you have been traveling has not always been an easy one. What's more, the journey is not over. Far from it. As you are discovering, there is always the need to learn more and to keep on growing.

Now that you are well on your life journey, you've probably begun to develop some perspective, and can step back a little to gauge what you've done right and what you've done wrong, what your strengths and weaknesses are, and what's important and what isn't. The important elements of our life journeys are stamina, energy, commitment, and passion. Chances are, you've always had the passion. Your interest in beauty and fashion may have set you apart from your peers at first. You probably dressed with more style than they did, which made you different. But in time, your friends started to turn to you for fashion advice, then maybe looked to you for advice about a whole range of life issues.

Your interest in beauty and fashion has always gone hand in hand with your interest in people. Cosmetologists are like that. People are always telling you things, confiding in you, trusting you. Whether you are quiet or outgoing, funny or serious, impulsive or organized, somehow you have this quality that draws people to you.

As you grew older, that perspective started to kick in and you began to learn things about yourself. Your interest became a focus and your focus became a goal. That explains why you are sitting here now, reading this book. You sailed off on your life journey, and even though you may have gotten stuck in the shallows sometimes or felt like you were being tossed by gales, you stuck it out. Did you have a mentor to help you? A family member perhaps, or an older friend or cosmetology professional who recognized your interest and saw your potential? Did that person direct you toward a future in cosmetology? Or did you do it all on your own, going up against the resistance of a mother or a father who thought that being a teacher or a doctor or a lawyer was a better choice for you?

It may even have been downright scary when you made up your mind to become a cosmetologist. For one thing, it meant making a serious investment in yourself and you had to ask yourself if you were worth it. Or maybe you were out in the world already, working at a job that didn't feel all that special but that still provided you with a regular paycheck. Giving that up was a giant decision. Going to cosmetology school would mean juggling things—your finances, and the demands on your personal time, to name two—and you weren't sure how great a juggler you would turn out to be.

Take finances, for instance. Imagine that you had saved up a tidy sum so that you could make a special trip. Were you ready to trade in long walks on the beach and piña coladas for beauty school tuition? You may have faced an even harder decision if you needed to borrow money. Who were you going to go to? Family? Friends? Were there going to be strings attached and what kind of strings would they turn out to be?

Everywhere you turned there were problems that needed to be addressed. If you had a spouse and kids, you had to figure out how you were going to meet their needs at the same time you were going to pursue this great adventure in your life. As you were to find out, there were no easy answers. It all had to do with your determination and your will to make this plan of action happen.

As you suspected, getting through cosmetology school was no picnic. Do you remember when you had to memorize all that stuff about disulfide bonds and salt bonds, and voltage and amperes? Today, these things probably come to you like second nature, but when you first saw them, they might just as well have been in another language. But you applied yourself, and the more you did, the more you became fascinated with the intricacies and challenges of the cosmetology profession.

Going from school to the real world was also a challenge, even if you already had plenty of real-world experience under your belt before going into cosmetology. It felt like a big difference being in a profession and not just doing a job. But after all, you had invested a great deal in this profession and you understandably wanted a good return of your investment. So you worked hard to present yourself in the very best light to future employers. You spiffed up your résumé and brushed up on your interviewing skills. You did the legwork to find which salons were in the area of your job search, and you took the time to consider and decide if you would be happiest in a small independent salon, a chain salon, a value-priced salon, or maybe even a day spa.

If you were lucky, your first job went well and you may still be in it. People were supportive, and there was plenty of opportunity to learn and to stretch. If you were not so lucky, there were some problems on that first job. The boss was unreadable, or the staff was overworked and competitive with each other, or there was a major style gulf between you and the clientele, or business was too slow. So you viewed that first job strictly as a résumé-builder, putting the best spin on it that you could, and you got out at the right time. The second job was better, the third was good, and since then, even though there have been hitches here and there, you have been able to enjoy the fruits of what is known as "progress."

Things have been so good that maybe you've even been able to realize a whole other dream, one that you may not have even had in sight at the beginning: to strike out on your own. Perhaps you started in a contained and conservative way by renting a booth in an established salon. Or maybe you and an associate got backing from private investors and opened up a salon of your own. And it's going well, even though you've never worked so hard in your life.

Whatever you've done in your career as a cosmetologist and whatever your route has been to get there, as a member in good standing of this amazing profession, you will be able to relate to many of the stories told here by your fellow cosmetologists and will be able to benefit from the helpful hints that we have collected.

The majority of cosmetologists we talked to truly love this profession and cite the following reasons.

◉ The ongoing creative challenge.

◉ The independent, self-starting aspect of the work that is present at every level in this field.

◉ The income opportunities realized right from the start.

◉ The possibilities for entrepreneurship, not only in terms of the long-range dream of owning one's own business but also in terms of retailing opportunities that are available along the way.

◉ The connections to people as a member of the salon team and the relationships one develops with one's clientele.

◉ The mobility of this "go-anywhere" profession and the fact that if you wish to move from

Dayton to Honolulu, chances are you will always be able to find a job.

◎ The satisfaction that comes with helping people look their best. All the cosmetologists talked about the joy of seeing the smile on their clients' faces when they went off to special occasions—a wedding, a prom, a graduation, a big interview—looking their absolute best.

The cosmetologists we spoke with also shared a keen awareness of the pitfalls and problems that are built into their work. Some that were cited include:

◎ falling into the trap of doing things the same way all the time, so that work runs the risk of becoming stale and uninspired.

◎ dealing with difficult personalities whether they are your boss, your coworkers, or your clients.

◎ losing the balance between your personal and professional lives, and falling prey to workaholism, procrastination, burnout, and other kinds of unproductive behaviors.

◎ having difficulty managing the physical demands of the work including the stress involved in a typical workday, and the strains on the body from chronic wear and tear.

How can men and women working in the cosmetology profession manage to hold onto the good feelings while dealing effectively with the drawbacks and negative feelings? For starters, they can learn from each other. No one is better equipped to offer support and advice to cosmetologists than other cosmetologists who are out there, in the field, discovering on a day-to-day basis what works and what doesn't.

This book is a compilation of hints, tips, and advice from cosmetologists all over the country. As writers, we gathered this information and then organized it in a way that we thought would be useful, but we never tampered with the information. We are not cosmetology experts. We are the channel through which you will hear from the experts.

The nitty-gritty advice that fills this book, however, needs to be placed in the context of broader, more sweeping principles. We have developed these principles during the course of writing Survival Guides for professionals in a number of different fields. The Seven Principles that you are about to learn are designed to help you determine what you value most in your life and how you can make room for the things you most value.

Seven Guiding Principles

Once you've read through these principles, it is important to keep them firmly in your mind. Post them on the wall by your station, keep them in your wallet, or write them on an index card and put it in your bag. If you want, you can turn them into a poem or a song and chant them at quiet times or, ritually, once a day, in the morning, perhaps, or before you go to sleep. The goal is to develop a healthy perspective that will sustain you over the long run, that will enable you to have fun and enjoy life, and that will help you remember—at the end of a day—what it is that you love about your work.

Principle #1: Become an Active Listener

If you have found yourself in the cosmetology field, the likelihood is that you are a "people person" and that you've always been a good listener. But whether you are or not, we can all do with a refresher course when it comes to listening. Here and elsewhere in this book, you will find specific tips on techniques like reflective listening in which you reinforce what people say by returning their questions and comments to them. As a guiding principle, we stress the importance of taking time in a busy day to listen to others and really hear what they have to say. Many of us are so overwhelmed by the demands and stresses of our work and personal lives that we look for relief by drowning out our surrounding environment, and tuning out others by becoming insensitive and oblivious to what they have to say. In fact, this drowning-out process intensifies stress. You can better attain stress relief by keeping open the lines of communication, and enjoying the contact and camaraderie that is always a potential in your relationships with staff and clients. Keep in mind, however, that by communication we mean the act of engaging with others in real dialogue: that is, saying what you have to say and actively listening to what comes back to you.

Principle #2: Thinking Outside the Box

Life will be a lot more satisfying if you avoid the trap of conventional, unimaginative, stereotyped thinking. One of the challenges you may be facing as a cosmetologist might have to do with being asked to style hair in a way that does not appeal to your own sense of aesthetics. If this is the case, you will need to find ways to keep your creativity alive and fresh outside of your job and outside of the box. You may want to spend one or two evenings a week styling the hair of friends whose taste is as dynamic as your own. Thinking outside the box will also help you to avoid stereotypical thinking that has to do with body image. This kind of thinking is not only wrong and can get you into a lot of trouble, but also deprives you of really meaningful opportunities you could be enjoying with others. Having an expansive, long-range view of things is another way of thinking outside the box. You may feel stuck in a rut right now, but you need to keep your dreams alive and know that life is always filled with surprises that might take you to places you never even imagined.

Principle #3: Take Time to Figure Out What You Find Most Satisfying

Well-organized systems and routines can help ensure smooth sailing for cosmetologists such as yourself, but routines can be overdone as well. When this happens, you may begin to feel like a robot, moving through your day without really thinking about what you're doing.

Mihaly Cziksentmihalyi, Ph.D., Professor of Psychology at the Drucker School of Management at Clermont Graduate University, did a study with adolescents where he outfitted them with beepers that went off eight times a day over the course of one week each year. Every time the beeper signaled, they'd report in to him about what they were doing and how they were feeling about it. Among other things, he found that when people are involved in an activity they enjoy, they develop a sense of *flow*, a great feeling of energy that makes them want to continue doing what they're doing and return to it whenever possible.

In Chapter 2, we will offer a tool and a technique to help you figure out which activities give you a sense of flow. We will help you assess how you spend your time and how you feel about what you're doing. We will take you through your day—before, after, and during work—and analyze where you feel most and least satisfied. This kind of honest assessment is a critical step you need to take before moving on to Principle #4.

Principle #4: Create Time for the Things You Care About

The idea of shifting your time and energies to accommodate the things you most enjoy may seem like common sense, but you would be surprised how few people actually live by this principle. Too many of us carry around a "can't do" attitude when it comes to changing our patterns. The good news is that most of us "can do" this kind of alteration.

Suppose you discover that you feel most ready to meet your workday after you have had thirty minutes of quiet time to sit, read the paper, and sip your coffee. Or perhaps you can achieve a better mood for the day if you've been able to take a walk before work begins. You may learn that by shifting morning chores with your spouse and children, you can free up the time you need. Or you might decide to set your alarm a half-hour earlier every day.

With regard to work, you may discover that the best way to do your paperwork is to collect it all and address it at the end of the day. On the other hand, you might find it easier to do the paperwork on the go. Each person's preference will be different. The key is to begin thinking about how you can best meet your needs because when your needs are met, you will be better equipped to meet the needs of others.

Principle #5: Learn to Enjoy What's in Front of You

There is a Buddhist practice called "mindfulness" that teaches the value of focusing on what is beautiful in the here and now. Mindfulness advocates living in the moment, and learning to develop this kind of vision is a huge help in clearing away the clutter in our lives.

How often have you found yourself thinking about everything other than what you are doing? You may be sitting in a staff meeting and your mind is wandering to your bills, that worrisome school conference you had about your child, the bad wheezy sound coming out of your car, or a million other things. Think about what it would be like to really focus in on the moment and get the most out of that meeting. Your colleagues and boss are all smart people who have many worthwhile things to say. *You* have many worthwhile things to say, too, and your active participation will go a long way toward making the salon a better environment.

This practice of mindfulness can and should be used outside of work, too. When you're driving home, for instance, instead of thinking about your bills, the worrisome school conference, or the weird sound in the car, think instead about how beautiful the light in the sky looks at that very moment or how peaceful the rain on your rooftop sounds.

Principle #6: Learn to be Flexible

There is no such thing as a day that goes exactly according to plan. You have to learn to roll with the punches and the bumps, and the trap doors that are always opening up all over the place. Cosmetology is a field particularly filled with the unexpected. Clients can either call at the last minute (or not call at all) to cancel appointments, or they may have emergencies when they simply have to see you. As part of a team, you may also be called on to fill in for someone else at the last minute.

If you think of yourself as a kind of machine out there every day getting the job done, then flexibility can be the lubricant that keeps your gears in working order. Stress is vanquished in the face of flexibility and flexibility also softens the hard edges that can often be present in one's interactions with others. Flexibility will keep you from turning into a tight rubber band, ready to snap. It serves as a strong and pliable elastic that allows you to retain your shape.

Principle #7: Prioritize

Once you know what you have to do and what you *love* to do, it's time to prioritize and get rid of all the unnecessary, energy-sapping tasks that you dread. You'll be shocked by how much choice you have about where to invest your efforts. Remember to keep track of what you actually do with your time. Ask yourself:

◉ "What do I need to do to take care of myself that absolutely no one else can do?" For example, "Do I need to meditate at the end of a long day after having dealt with the needs of other people?" Or, "Do I need to make dinner plans with others from the salon to cement my working relationships with them?"

◉ "Which of my responsibilities can be put off for the moment so that I can deal with them later with no harm done?" For example, "Can I take care of my promotional activities (sending out cards to clients, let's say) at home? Can I come in early tomorrow and inventory my supplies instead of trying to do it on this busy day?"

◉ "What am I doing that someone else could be doing for me? Am I making full use of our assistants and interns? To do so would not only help me but could very well help them."

Embodying these Seven Guiding Principles and letting them show you the way is not something that happens overnight. Some people take months, even years, before they can internalize them, and, even then, most of us have to be vigilant about not letting our counterproductive habits creep back into control. As time goes on, these principles will come to feel like second nature, and when you fully understand them and live by them, you will appreciate and enjoy a quality of life you might never have experienced otherwise.

Chapter Reference

Cziksentmihalyi, M. (1991). *The psychology of optimal experience.* New York: HarperCollins.

Chapter 2

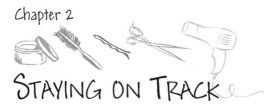

STAYING ON TRACK

Generally, when people say to us, "How are you doing?" we answer "Fine." That's just the way it is. We don't really expect people to be interested in what was bad or good about our day. But in that kind of ongoing exchange—*"How are you doing?" "Fine."*—something often gets lost along the way. The details of our day become blurred. We run the risk of becoming almost as uninterested and unattentive to what is going on in our lives as the people who keep asking us that same hollow question.

In this book, we suggest that you give some serious thought to how you view your day. The best way to begin is by keeping a record of the way you use your time. Most of us spend 16 out of every 24 hours a day awake and active. That's on a good day. Unfortunately, for some of us, the waking day stretches out to 18 or 19 hours. In those waking hours, some of what we do makes us feel great. We are kept busy with activities that leave us feeling energized and happy, with that sense of flow that we cited in the first chapter. But, unfortunately, all of us have to spend some of those waking hours doing things we would rather not be doing; things that are boring or unpleasant, or that we even dread.

In many instances, we don't have much choice about much of what we have to do. With rare exceptions, most people are faced with the need to do some of the humdrum activities of life such as paying bills, doing the laundry, and going grocery shopping. Sometimes, it feels relentless and laborious. But it is our belief that most of us actually have more control over our lives than we give ourselves credit for. The key is to begin to think about what it is that we do with our time and to keep track of our feelings with regard to these activities. Once we've done that, we can begin to think about making changes.

This book is very focused on how to simplify and improve the professional lives of cosmetologists. To that end, however, it is important that you explore the ways in which you spend your time, not only at work, but also before and after work. There is a direct emotional link from one sphere of your life to the other.

One stylist named Jan, who worked at a day spa, told us how she'd gotten into this habit of coming home from work every night, fixing dinner for her family, and then collapsing in front of whatever was on television. "It was ironic," she said. "Here I was, working in this gorgeous environment, with everything geared to teaching people how to achieve the best quality of life and how to make the strongest kind of mind-body connection, and it was all rolling off me like water off a duck's back. I was so overtired that the only thing I could think about was vegging out."

A friend of Jan's persuaded her to join a class on Film Appreciation at a local community college. "I didn't want to at first, but my friend, who sells phone systems, doesn't take no for an answer. So I went," Jan said. "We'd meet twice a week, watch a great movie like *Chinatown* or *Thelma and Louise*, and have a really good discussion afterward."

The class was a revelation for Jan for whom the idea of going out at night during the week had been unimaginable. "I just loved the class," she said. "The fact is I always wanted to be an actress.

I did a lot of theater work when I was younger and even had a few bit parts in movies when I lived in Los Angeles. That's more or less how I got into styling. I appreciated the theatrical flavor of it. So to sit there watching a film at night followed by an intelligent discussion was just such a treat and such a welcome change from eating Butter Brickle ice cream out of the carton in front of the television. Even though I was getting less sleep than usual because of the class (I'd been in the habit of getting into bed by nine, and on film nights didn't get home till eleven), I still felt much more energized."

Jan came to realize that when you spend your days catering to the needs of other people, you often run out of juice when it comes to taking care of your own needs. It is crucial that you make time to tend to your spouse or partner, your children, your extended family, your friends, and, last but hardly least, yourself. You need to set aside time to cultivate your outside interests, your hobbies, and all the facets that go into making you a multifaceted person.

This is not to say that there is anything wrong with sitting in front of the television with Butter Brickle ice cream. There is a time and a place for everything, and our purpose in this book is not to pass judgment or set down rules. If sitting in front of the television and vegging out is what you need to do to relax, then go with it. But if it leaves you somehow feeling even more tired and drained, if it actually saps you of your energy as that kind of passive activity can tend to do, then it is time to find another kind of release.

 Keeping Track

In order to develop an awareness of how you feel about the way you are spending your time, you need to do some work. The pages that follow in this chapter make up a workbook of sorts. Look at the headings of the sections that follow.

◎ Start/Stop/Total

◎ Activity

◎ Feelings

◎ Efficiency

◎ What's My Role?

Copy them into a notebook that you can carry with you throughout the day. A small, spiral-bound pad will fit into almost any coat or jacket pocket for easy access.

Ideally, you will be creating a journal or log that reflects exactly what you do with your time in the course of any given day. This technique works especially well if you stay at it for a full week. Keeping track of your weekend activities and the feelings they engender can provide an interesting contrast to the study you make of your workweek habits.

It may be difficult for you to take the few minutes necessary to log activities. When you've got clients backed up and paperwork to attend to, not to mention that training seminar you have to somehow fit into your day, it isn't easy to find the time to make notes about your feelings. Just do the best you can to jot down the notes while the experience is still fresh in your mind. If you can glance at your watch and make a mental note of the time you begin and end an activity, you can always jot it down later.

Some people find it easier to make notes on a small tape recorder or dictation machine, the kind busy executives use to keep track of their thoughts. Do whatever works for you and do it as well as you can. The idea is not to create another burden in your life but to help you develop a powerful sense of awareness regarding the way you spend your time.

Let us have a look at the categories you will be keeping track of.

Start/Stop/Total

In this phase of taking stock, you will need to be conscious of the clock, right from the moment your alarm goes off in the morning until you close your eyes at night. Think about the distinct areas into which your activities fall: client consultation, hair-styling, sanitation and maintenance, staff interaction, scheduling, and so on. Check the clock when you begin one new activity and jot down the time. Do the same when you finish that activity and before you move on to the next one. Don't neglect to factor in things like "conferencing with staff" and the like. Just a few minutes spent with a colleague discussing a client can legitimately be considered conferencing. Whatever you do, don't worry about the total time spent until later. You don't need to burden yourself with adding, subtracting, and justifying yourself in the middle of a busy day.

Activity

This is where you will note what category your activity falls into. The more specific you are, the more you'll learn from this log at the end of the week. If you are consulting with a client on a new style she's considering for a friend's wedding, make a note of it. If you are involved in a staff meeting to figure out why so much waste is going on in the salon, make a note of it.

You will also want to examine the activity closely and pay attention to the kinds of interactions that go into it. For instance, in the case of a consultation, do you start out with a casual, catching-up exchange? Do you have your style scrapbook at the ready or are you hunting around for it? Do you spend quality time looking through haircolor swatches and hearing your client's input?

Everything that is a part of your day should find its way into your log. And remember, this is not something you'll be graded on. You are the sole creator, contributor, and judge of what is included, and you are the only one who will read it. The goal is to learn about yourself: how you spend your time and how you feel about yourself during the course of a day.

Cosmetologists work in a high-stress job. Many demands are made on them and the work is physically taxing. Maintaining this log should never feel like an additional burden. The goal is to make your life easier, and despite the extra effort this will require—for a short period at least—it will ultimately go a long way toward meeting that goal. Hang in there and do the best you can with it.

Feelings

Try to jot down your feelings soon after you have finished an activity. The closer you are to the feelings, the less likely you will be to edit them, either consciously or unconsciously. Keep in mind that you do not need to write long, detailed notes here. A few words, if well chosen, will do fine. Begin by thinking in terms of feeling words such as happy, sad, angry, bored, or worried. More clarification might come by thinking in terms of opposites—happy/sad, relaxed/tense, worried/optimistic, loving/angry, gentle/tough, energetic/tired, interested/bored—and seeing to which of the two poles in each instance you feel closer.

It is also important in this section to gauge how much satisfaction you are getting out of your activities. Most of us have to do things that are not necessarily fun, but aspects of these activities can still give us a deep sense of satisfaction. If you are a very tactile person, for instance, which you probably are given that you have chosen cosmetology as your profession, you probably get a certain sense of satisfaction from spreading a fragrant, luxurious emollient on a thick head of hair. If you are a people person, the time you spend catching up with a favorite customer probably is a great source of satisfaction in your day. You may be the kind of person who can relieve the burden of a laborious task just by having music on the radio or by focusing in on the beauty of a bouquet of anemones you are keeping at your workstation.

Once you figure out what it is that gives you pleasure and a sense of well-being, you'll be in a better position to think about how you can adjust your schedule to make the most of those activities and make the least of the ones you don't find satisfying. This might require swapping responsibilities with fellow workers, but, then again, they might love doing what you like least. Some people, for instance, like nothing more than to organize a messy drawer or closet.

Remember not to think too hard and too long when you write down your reactions. Your gut response is probably the most reliable. Again, keep in mind that this log is for your eyes only. Don't worry about what others will think of you when you put down your honest reactions. This log is a tool that exists only to make your life simpler and more pleasant. As we said above, it is not something on which you are going to be graded.

Efficiency

Chances are you know someone who is a marvelous hairstylist but who cannot ever get through a job without forgetting where some important tool or material was placed. Maybe you are such a person. With this log, you will be keeping close tabs on your efficiency quotient.

Keep in mind that efficiency is not the absolute highest ideal in the world. We have all known people who are incredibly efficient and those who aren't. Where do you fall? Do you freak out if your hairpins aren't lined up neatly in a row? If someone moves something of yours, do you turn on the siren and put out an all-points bulletin? Are you the sort who is continuously raiding other people's supplies? Does your station look like a whirlwind blew through it? Is your bag bulging at the seams with equal weight given to important things like a client's business card, and the trivial like an expired coupon to a car wash in a neighborhood you almost never visit? The point of the log is to look at the matter of efficiency—how best to use your time—and to strike a balance that is comfortable for you and the people with whom you work and live.

There will be many instances in the log where efficiency really is not all that relevant. For example, if you are looking at the time of day when you cook dinner, you may find that you don't necessarily choose to be as efficient as possible. While you might have a food processor that could do the job of chopping vegetables much faster than you can by hand, perhaps on that particular evening, you are drawing a certain contemplative comfort from doing the task by hand, enjoying the feel of the vegetables and the steady slice of the knife. Maybe that is just the medicine you need to bring you down from a stressful day. So, if efficiency does not apply to a given task, simply write NA (meaning not applicable) in your log. Otherwise, make an effort to rate your efficiency in any given activity on a scale of 1 to 5.

What's My Role?

In the three-act play called *A Day in Your Life*, one plays a host of roles over the course of 24 hours. The person may be parent, child, spouse, partner, manager, confidante, taskmaster, mentor, confessor, social worker, or whatever. You name it. It is useful to think about which roles you most enjoy and which suit you best. Compile a list, somewhere in the back of your notebook or pad, of all the roles you play over the course of a given week. Use it as a reference when you make your log entries.

When you get up in the morning, think about the many roles that you will be playing that day. As you fill in your log, figure out the role that you have been playing for that activity, but you don' t necessarily have to write it down then and there. This category and the next—End-of-Day Analysis—can be filled in at the end of the day when you find some quiet time for reflection.

	Activity #1	Activity #2	Activity #3
Start			
Stop			
Total			
Feelings			
Efficiency			
What's My Role			

 End-of-Day Analysis

Now for the fun! The very last thing you do each day just before you turn out the lights is to analyze your log. This is your opportunity to learn something about yourself, and believe it or not, for many people, the results are genuinely surprising. Follow the steps below.

1. Begin by totaling the first column, Start/Stop/Total. Add up the total for each activity and note it.

2. Review what you've written in the Activity column and read down the row to What's My Role? Think about what your role has been in each activity and note it in the appropriate place.

3. When you've filled in the entire What's My Role? column, check back to the Feelings column and think about which roles you found most pleasurable or satisfying. Note as well those activities that you found least pleasurable or satisfying. Give yourself time to think about how you might rearrange your life to maximize your time spent in the pleasurable roles and minimize the time spent in those roles you do not enjoy.

4. Look back at your Start/Stop/Total column and match it up against the Feelings column. How much time did you spend doing things that offered you very little satisfaction? How much time did you get to spend doing the things you most love to do?

5. Think about what was most surprising in your log and make a note of it. Perhaps it was how much time you spent doing things that you genuinely did not enjoy. Or maybe—hopefully—it was the other way around. Maybe you're surprised by how much

pleasure you take in being a manager of people. Maybe you are surprised by how little pleasure you get from actually being behind the chair working on a client's hair.

6. Repeat this process every day for a week, each day with a new log. At the end of the week, go over all your notes, paying special attention to the End-of-the-Day Analysis. Give yourself ample time to think about what you are reading.

Again, the goal here is to reflect. Ultimately, you will want to find enough time in your life to do more of what you love to do and less of what you don't like to do. In order to achieve that goal, you will need to keep track of the Seven Guiding Principles.

1. Become an active listener.

2. Think outside of the box.

3. Take time to figure out what you find most satisfying.

4. Create time for the things you care about.

5. Learn to enjoy what is in front of you.

6. Learn to be flexible.

7. Prioritize.

Keeping a log and being mindful of the Seven Guiding Principles is only one step toward simplifying your life as a cosmetologist, however. The next step involves absorbing the shortcuts and tips you will be hearing from your fellow cosmetologists. This way, you can learn from others how to make room for the things you most enjoy.

Chapter 3

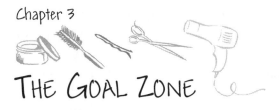

THE GOAL ZONE

A s we have said elsewhere in this book, cosmetology is a highly demanding profession. The talents it calls on are multidimensional. As a cosmetologist, your first task is to deal with people. You have to be able to hear what they tell you, and in return, you have to get them to hear you. In any service profession, you deal with a wide range of personalities, and people may not be that sensitive to your feelings or needs. And we're not talking only about clients. Unless you are working for yourself, you will be dealing with coworkers as part of a team. Even if you own your own business, you still need real people skills. You will have to learn how to manage and motivate others, which can sometimes be harder than motivating yourself and managing your own time.

A cosmetologist needs to be technically adroit, creative, and invested in continuing education. The developments in technology in the beauty industry are ongoing, and the learning curve never straightens out. As a cosmetologist, you will need energy, stamina, and grit to help you carry your workload, and to keep you fresh and active. You will also want to develop sufficient resources to keep you from burning out from stress and overload.

If you are a cosmetologist with ambitions to own your own business or even to operate a booth rental, you will need to develop as good a business head as you can. You will want to have a basic working knowledge of budgeting, taxes, how to read a balance sheet, and handle important financial matters like that. At the very least, you will need people to help you—a bookkeeper or an accountant—so that you make the most of your finances.

If you are a seasoned pro in this business, you already know a lot of the above. If you're still a relative newcomer, you are making your way through a lot of these issues. In either case, you should always be setting goals for yourself. An important aspect of goal-setting has to do with your definition of success. Let's look at what your peers are saying on that subject.

The Fundamentals of Success

Success works best when it is part of a world-view. It is not the pot of gold at the end of the rainbow, but, rather, an organic element in the way you see the world and your role in it.

◎ Lots of people think that success is all about how much money you make. It's so much more than that. To me, success is about the life skills you can claim. Are you genuinely helpful and caring to other people? Can you stick to a job and see it through to completion? Are you a substantial, competent human being, or just a lucky one who happened to be in the right place at the right time?

◎ To me, success hinges on how much patience you have. If you work hard and have basic skills and talent, *and* if you're patient and are willing to hang in there for the long haul, chances are you'll get your rewards.

◎ People will tell you that success is all about who you know. In a sense, that's correct, but not in such a cynical way. To me, "who you know" means making yourself available to people. Enjoying people with all their strengths and weaknesses is key to this business.

◎ When I think of success, I think of *adaptation*. Sure, anybody can be a winner in the best of situations. But how do you fare when the going gets tough? What do you do when you're in a sub-par work situation, with shoddy facilities and people who are not necessarily out to protect your best interests? The ability to navigate a rough situation and come out of it intact is probably a better indicator of future success than anything else.

⦿ When young people ask me how to become successful, I always start with organization. I'm sorry, but neatness counts. When I see someone with a bag that's overflowing with junk or a work area that looks dirty and unkempt, I cross that person off my list. Not forever! Just until she can get her act together.

⦿ Some people become successful without a sense of humor, but I don't know how they do it. I certainly couldn't have survived in this business without one. Crazy clients? I make fun of them (but only to myself!) I make fun of me, too. Whenever I do something stupid, I'm the first one to point it out. Always beat your colleagues to the punch when it comes to criticism. Steal the fire, I say.

⦿ The characteristic that I've found in common with most successful people I know is that they see the big picture. They don't allow themselves to get bogged down in details. If they need help, they ask for it. Successful people learn what they need to know, and disregard what's irrelevant.

◎ I've known many talented, ambitious people who fall short of success. You know why? Because they lack common sense. You'd be amazed how many smart people lack common sense. You see it particularly in the way people relate to other people. I've seen people I thought were smart chew out a customer for being late. Does that make sense?

◎ I've been asked to mentor a lot of people over the years. Sometimes it's worked out, sometimes not. One warning signal for me is when I'm involved with a person who doesn't really see things through to completion. For instance, they'll do 92 percent of a cleanup. Everything is really nice and neat except that they don't bother to put the lids back on the jars. Now you might think that's just a little thing, but to me, it's a mind-set. It's all about resistance, and often it's about resistance to success.

◎ What is success? People will tell you that it's money and maybe independence. Sure, those things are important, but they don't tell the whole story. You absolutely cannot be a successful person, by my terms anyway, unless you're an ethical person. Success is all about a way of looking at life, and I don't want to be involved with anyone who looks at life without a clear sense that ethics is a large part of the picture.

◎ A good hint for maintaining a successful frame of mind is to tell yourself that you're special. Everyone is special. Everyone has a set of gifts and talents that is as unique as a fingerprint. Some people, for instance, have such an incredibly defined sense of smell that they are hired by perfume manufacturers to be "sniffers." Now that's a special gift that I imagine took a while for the person to figure out he had. We all have to take the time to figure out what our special gifts are. But they're there, all right.

◎ Success is fueled by passion. It's best when the passion is for the thing you do, whether you have a passion for art or music or sports or hairstyling. Some people succeed, however, because they simply have a passion for success. They see themselves as being successful and so they become successful.

◎ My father, bless his heart, taught me that there is no such thing as failure. Every action has a result. Some are good, some are bad. When it's a bad result, that's all it is: a bad result. It's not a catastrophe. It's not a disaster. It's not the end of the world. Just put the best face on it and turn it into a learning experience.

◎ Success is beautiful, success is great, but even more important is self-validation. To know that you are a good, worthwhile human being even without success is to be truly successful.

 ## Guidelines for Success

Hundreds of how-to books have been written that offer prescriptions for success. The general consensus is that success has to do with hard work, talent, and luck. But there are some specific guidelines to keep in mind when you are going after success. Here are some tips from your colleagues in the field.

◎ Don't even think about achieving success if you don't have a strong sense of self-esteem. If you're lucky, you can build on a base of self-esteem that began in your childhood. Some of us are not so lucky, however, and have to undo the lessons we learned about being bad, lazy, stupid, or worthless. Self-esteem kicks in when you allow yourself to have good feelings about the things you do. And not just the work things. Let yourself feel good about the omelet you cooked, about the plant you've kept alive, about the exercise routine you maintain, about the kindness you've showed a friend, and about the loving person you are to your own family.

◎ A really important technique to help you achieve success is *visualization*. Athletes use visualization all the time. They see themselves hitting a ball or crossing a finish line, and seeing makes for believing. If you see yourself as a successful person who is on top of things and is interacting effectively with other people, then you can begin to turn those possibilities into realities.

⊚ Success is great and everyone wants it, but guess what? Everyone doesn't get it, and certainly it doesn't always come easily. Life is full of hurdles. Sometimes, success seems to be right there at your fingertips, only to slip through at the last minute. So the best way to ultimately be successful is to be kind to yourself. Don't wear yourself out with criticism and self-recrimination. Everyone makes mistakes. Everyone is unlucky at one time or another. Preserve your good feelings about yourself by being good to yourself, and you'll survive until success is ready to visit you.

⊚ Take care of yourself physically, emotionally, mentally, and spiritually. Even if you become successful, you're not going to stay that way unless you're vigilant about taking care of yourself. I've seen plenty of one-shot wonders burn themselves out. Don't eat, sleep, and drink work. Take time out for family, friends, exercise, and the relaxed enjoyment of life.

⊚ Define success for yourself. It's your life and you should be the judge of what is or what is not successful. Maybe your father thought that success meant making at least $50,000 a year. Maybe your mother defined success as marrying a rich doctor. Those are their worldviews. What is right for your father or your mother or your brother or your uncle is not necessarily right for you.

◎ I like to think of success as something you can get good at. And the way to get good at it is to first get good at a lot of the habits that lead to success. To me, that means good posture, good hygiene, being well dressed, speaking with confidence and clarity, using good grammar, practicing polite manners by doing things like sending thank-you notes when it is appropriate, and so on. All of this creates a positive self-image that can go a long way toward ushering in success.

◎ I can't overemphasize the importance of pacing yourself. That means getting enough rest. There is nothing more important than that. Eating well. Spending quality time with your friends and family. Exercising. Success can take a long time in coming. If you wear yourself out going at it in a dogged way, you might not only miss out on the success but also on everything else that life has to offer.

◎ Always respect other people. If you truly believe in fair play and basic decency, you can avoid a lot of the mistakes that people make. Being deceitful or dismissive with anyone, even people you think you may never en-counter again or who have no obvious impor-tance in your life, can come back to haunt you and to spoil your plans.

◉ To me, the number one enemy of success is pro-crastination. We all do it, so it's not something to feel guilty about. It's just something to learn to overcome. Telling yourself that you're going to do it tomorrow is the worst mistake you can make. If you dread doing something—like study-ing for a huge exam, let's say—find some little bit of the task that you can separate out and start with that. Maybe it's sharpening pencils. Maybe it's organizing file cards. Whatever. Just don't ever allow yourself to become paralyzed.

◉ You might think that perfectionism is the spur to success but you'd be wrong. Perfectionism is a way to punish yourself. We all have bad days. That's life. Striving for perfection is a lot of foolishness and can only leave you with the constant bitter taste of disappointment. Who needs that?

Success Strategies That You Can Put into Place

In addition to the preceding guidelines, many of the cosmetologists we spoke to cited certain strategies that they felt were crucial to success: things like game plans and mission statements. These are the nuts and bolts that you can use to create a structure on which to build your success.

◎ Once you've decided what it is you want to do, then you need a game plan. I like to think of myself as a business. If I owned a business, which I plan to one day, I'd have to develop a business plan, right? It would be the blueprint that would get me from here to there. If I didn't have one, no one would lend me a cent. So, if I think of *myself* as a business. I can make a kind of business plan but instead I'll call it a game plan. It tells me where I want to be in a year, in two years, in five years, and maybe even in ten years.

◎ The important thing about a game plan, which I believe all people should have at every point in life, is that it tells you what kind of resources and training you'll need to get you where you want to go. If you're a student starting out in life, you need a game plan that will help you figure out where you're going to get your tuition money, where you're going to find a quiet place to study, how you can balance your life as a student with the job you need to hold down, and so forth. If you're a retiree, you need to have a plan to show you how you're going to live off your savings, how you're going to occupy your time to make you a happy and fulfilled person, and where you can live that's easy and convenient. Without a game plan, you're just whistling in the dark.

◎ You can't be successful without a strong sense of motivation. And motivation is strongly tied in to how happy you are. Someone taught me the 80/20 Rule: love 80 percent of what you do and accept the fact that the remaining 20 percent is going to be drudge work. Even if you have to work your around the clock to do that 80 percent part, you can still love it. Challenges and demands make life interesting. But when the balance goes out of whack—when the 20 percent goes up to 50 percent or even 80 percent—then you know it's time to reassess and to put a whole new game plan into action.

◎ I back up my game plan with a mission statement. If you ever look at a business plan, it always includes a mission statement. The mission statement defines who you are and identifies your long-term goals. It's amazing how helpful it is to see your life in such concrete terms.

◎ I write my mission statement on a business-size card that I then have laminated. What can I say? I'm a neatness freak. I then keep it in my wallet and pull it out and look at it. A lot. What it says is that I am committed to doing my best as I go through life. That's all I can do—my best—but my best is pretty darn good.

- I re-do my mission statement every six months or maybe once a year, depending on what comes up in my life. The goals change but the basic definition of who I am has basically stayed the same. "I am a person dedicated to living my life with dignity, honesty, and integrity." Now why would I want to change that?

- I have a lot of distractions in my life—two kids, an ex-husband who doesn't like to live up to his responsibilities, and a mother with chronic health problems—so it's really easy for me to get waylaid from my goals. A mission statement keeps me on track. I have four copies of my mission statement. I put one in my wallet, one on my bed table, one in the glove compartment of my car, and I keep one at work. I'm thinking of getting it tattooed on my forehead!

- A mission statement is not only for you; it's for your clients to see as well. I keep mine in a frame at work. Some of my clients have asked me, "Is that for real?" I tell them, "You bet it is."

- A very wise person I knew taught me the secret of "positive self-talk." I use it all the time, keeping up a dialogue with myself. When I do something well, I say to myself, "Good job." When I flub something, I say, "You gave it the old college try, kid." When I'm incredibly nervous about something, I actively help myself by saying, "You're a strong woman. You have what it takes. *I'm here for you.*"

Goal-Setting

◎ You've got to understand that there are goals and then there are goals. In other words, some goals are short term—you can realize them tomorrow or next week or in a couple of months—and some are goals for the long haul. Owning your own business, for instance, is, for most people, a long-term goal, unless maybe you've got a rich uncle.

◎ To me, a lot of long-term goals are more "feeling"-type goals. To feel financially secure. To be in a committed relationship with someone you love. To feel really good about yourself and free of that voice you grew up with telling you that you were a loser. Those goals may take a long time to achieve, but it can happen.

◎ Setting goals can become a totally counter-productive activity if you find that you keep falling short of them. In other words, if you can't meet your goals, you'll become disappointed and even discouraged, which doesn't help anybody. So what I do is I break down my goals, even my short-term ones, into smaller "goal units" that I know I can accomplish. For instance, when I was in cosmetology school, I was really worried in the beginning because, believe me, I'm no student. But I broke the whole experience down into a bunch of short-term goals—get your homework assignments done; pass your exams; master the techniques—and that made it all less overwhelming.

◎ When you're setting goals for yourself, keep in mind what you'll need in order to achieve them. Ask yourself questions like, "What skills do I need to reach my goal?" "Do I need to take more classes?" "Can I find a coach or a mentor to help me?"

◎ First and foremost: analyze your goals to make sure that they are within the realm of possibility. For instance, if you've got chronic back problems, you don't want to become a hair stylist on your feet all day. Or if you've got a problem with hand-eye coordination, don't set a goal for yourself of becoming a major league ball player.

◎ When it comes to setting goals, know what you're getting into. Do your homework. If your goal is to work in a day spa, then first spend some significant time in a day spa. Splurge and go as a client if you have to. See if that's really what you want or whether it's some kind of romanticized notion that doesn't have a basis in the reality of who you really are.

- Goal-setting never ends. It's not as if you get to the top of the heap and you're finished with goals. Just look at amazingly successful people and you'll see that they are always raising the bar higher.

Dealing with Disappointment

Goals are important, but just as important is coping with not meeting your goals. The way you deal with disappointment and failure is key to how successful you will be at getting through life.

- I've been fired twice. The first time, I carried on for weeks like it was a Greek tragedy. My family and friends got so sick of me it wasn't even funny. The second time, I let my friends take me out to dinner. I had two Black Russians, I cried, and I got on with my life. That's called growing up.

- I think goals and game plans are great, and I would never in a million years warn anybody against them. But you have to understand that in the nature of reaching goals is the fact that you might fall short. My way of dealing with this is to look for the gift. That's kind of a Buddhist concept, as I understand it. It's saying that in every event, even in very bad ones, there is some kind of gift that will lead you to greater self-awareness. For instance, the first time I took my licensing exam, I failed it. I was shattered, but at the next exam, I wound up talking to another girl and we just had this instant click. We've been friends ever since. And that's what I mean by the "gift."

◉ Disappointments can lead you down streets you wouldn't have encountered otherwise. I was working at a salon that went under. It was no surprise but I wasn't motivated to get out and find another job until this happened. It took me a little while but I found a great job that I was in for six years. The bad news turned into good news.

A Delicate Balance

In going after your goals, it's important to strike that balance between too much and too little. Let's have a look at how others manage.

◉ I put the bar high. That's just who I am. I believe in continually trying to better myself. I never stop taking courses. I never rest on my laurels. I see myself as a work in progress.

◉ I try to pace myself. When I was younger, all I did was work. It was kind of a macho thing. The more I worked, the more powerful I felt. I ruined a lot of relationships that way.

- When you're in your own business, you run the risk of seeing yourself as a kind of money machine. The more hours you put in, the more money you can make. I know self-employed stylists who work 16-hour days!

- I take two vacations a year, no matter what. Even if I'm not having a very good year, I still take my vacations. Sometimes I'll stay at home, but I don't clean out closets or paint the back room. I do special things that I don't normally get to do. I might go to a movie in the afternoon. I might sit for an hour staring at a statue in a museum. Maybe I'll go to a botanical garden and study the shape of flowers. Some of my best vacations have been spent that way.

- In my experience, workaholics don't actually get more done than normal people. It's a mystery, but it's the truth. A lot of them are just sort of obsessive-compulsive personalities who take a lot more time doing simple or even unnecessary tasks just so that they can say they're working. Work is their drug of choice and, like any drug, work can be badly abused.

- One way I try to achieve a sense of balance between my professional and personal lives is by being part of a support group. For years now, I've been part of a group of women like myself. There are five of us: all stylists, all mothers, all trying to do their best to hold everything together. We have dinner one Friday a month. I can't tell you how much we all look forward to it. Sometimes we'll go out; sometimes we'll make a big pot of spaghetti at somebody's house. And then we'll just sit around, drink some wine, belly-ache, laugh, cry, or whatever. It makes such a difference knowing that you're not alone out there.

◎ I like to think I'm a balanced person, and one way I achieve that is making rules and living by them. For instance, I have a rule that I don't work past eight o'clock at night. My boss knows this about me and it's not an issue. At eight o'clock, I turn from Cinderella to a princess. I go to my dance class, I have dinner with friends, or I visit my aunt, who's housebound. I cultivate the other part of me. I won't give that up for anyone or anything.

◎ You know how some people train their kids not to bother them when they're work-ing? I do the opposite. I'm kind of a workaholic and I become obsessed when I'm taking a brush-up course or whatever. I tend to close out the world when I'm studying, so I've taught my kids to come in to me and say, "Ma, you're needed here. Hello? Earth to Ma." It works!

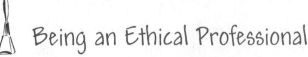

Being an Ethical Professional

A critical part of the mix that makes for success is a well-developed sense of ethics. Think of ethics as a code of conduct, teaching you to how to distinguish right from wrong. Ethics are the moral principles we live by. Without them, we can be led into dangerous and destructive places. With them, we have a compass to use on our journey through life. Here is how your colleagues in the field feel about ethics.

◎ There are ethical standards you have to adhere to as a cosmetologist. These are established by your state board. But ethics enter into your professional life in all kinds of ways such as how you interact with your clients and fellow employees or whether you are respectful and supportive. To act in a respectful and supportive way is to act in an ethical manner.

◎ I factor ethical behavior into my mission statement. I break it down into a number of characteristics and then I continually take an accounting of myself to make sure that I'm embodying those characteristics. For instance, I view ethical behavior as being honest above everything else. I think being attentive and punctual and cooperative are also aspects of ethical behavior. Other people might cite other characteristics but to me, those are the basic building blocks of my code of ethics.

- I've made "setting limits" a part of my ethical code. It's like learning to say no. If I know I can't do something—like work on a Saturday, let's say—I will make it known and I will stick to it. That way, everything is clear and above board, and no one's pretending they can do what they really can't do.

- I think ethics is an important issue in terms of the kind of success you can hope to have with a client. To me, it's a matter of ethics to really pay attention to my client, and to listen to the needs and desires that the client is trying to express. I feel I owe that to my client, and if I can't do that, then I'm not behaving in a professionally ethical manner.

- Ethics is a two-way street. A client has to know that it is unethical to cancel an appointment at the last minute and by making up some excuse, like the car won't start or a pipe burst. My pipes burst when I hear that!

- The one trait that is absolutely essential in order to reach and remain at the highest level of professionalism is commitment. An ethical person is committed to personal and professional growth. Ethical people don't coast along, don't take shortcuts, and don't take the easy way out.

- I equate ethics with integrity, and for me, one of the places that ethics really becomes an issue is around retailing. I regard it as highly unethical to sell a product I don't really believe in just to make a few bucks. On the other hand, I think it's truly ethical to source the best product for your client and to allow that client to spend her money or something that is really worth something.

◎ Ethics is really tied into success and here's an example. I knew a brilliant stylist with a blue-chip clientele who couldn't keep a confidence. He simply failed to understand that confidentiality is a foundation of ethical behavior for a cosmetologist. His clients would tell him things and he was continually indiscreet about not keeping these things to himself. The moral of the story is that he got caught, more than once, and you can be sure that he didn't hold on to his success.

◎ Not everyone would agree, but I think an ethical issue for a cosmetologist is the need to stay informed. Taking part in continuing education is, to me, a sign of sound ethics because it shows that you're committed to doing your very best for your client. And what could be more ethical than that?

Chapter 4

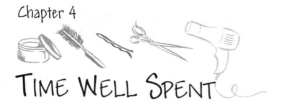

Time Well Spent

Until very recently, commuters in Boston, one of our nation's oldest cities, had to make their way along antiquated highways and roads that were really not up to today's standards. The city finally bit the bullet and initiated what came to be known as The Big Dig. This was a massive construction project that completely overhauled the city's infrastructure and brought it into the 21st century. It was hard for the town while the Big Dig was going on, but it was worth it.

Do you ever have the feeling that you've gotten a little bit like Boston? Are your roadways clogged and bottlenecked? Do things seem to take two or three times as long as they should? Do you find yourself either waiting or rushing? Do you tend to lose things a lot and then find them, sometimes literally under your nose? If all this sounds painfully familiar, then you might want to ask yourself if it's time to do a Big Dig of your own. Maybe you need to clear away debris, widen the lanes, design new routes, and bring yourself up to speed!

Getting organized and managing your time is part art, part science, and part pure determination. Even if it is not in your basic nature to be organized, you can still make significant improvements in that department. Consider the following tips from your fellow cosmetologists and start thinking about how you can put these ideas into practice.

Time Management

You've probably heard the expression, "Time heals all wounds." The issue of time certainly has the capacity to be wounding, frustrating, and confusing. People who are chronically late soon wear out the patience of others, and there are few professions as time-sensitive as cosmetology where you are asked to stick to a schedule that impacts on clients and coworkers. Cosmetologists who cannot manage their time run the risk of becoming cosmetologists with all the time in the world: in other words, out-of-work.

◎ The issue of time has always made me nervous. My father was like a drill sergeant. We couldn't even be three minutes late to church. My mother, on the other hand, had no sense of time whatsoever and I was forever waiting on street corners for her. So the whole time thing always made so nervous that I sought the help of a counselor who taught me about my "inner organizer." It's like a natural clock you carry around inside yourself. Some people have a quiet, measured clock; others have clocks that tick loud and fast. When you find out what your clock is like, you can learn to listen to it and let it guide you.

◎ Just because you're putting a time management system into place doesn't mean you're suddenly going to have to bustle around like some efficiency expert with a clipboard and a stopwatch. The point is for you to customize a system that reflects the way you like to live. Some people live by the clock whereas others need a more flexible system with blocs of "free time" set aside. That is not to say that these people can't be organized and efficient. It's just a question of style.

◎ For me, time management begins (and practically ends) with *prioritization*. Between my three teenagers and my high-stress job, I approach my day as if I'm part of a triage team trying to keep afloat in a flood. In other words, I have to figure out what I can do effectively, what I can try to do, and what I have to admit to myself that I simply can't do.

◉ A lot of people who have trouble with time management think of time as the enemy. They see time as the thing that is slipping away from them, that's being sucked down the hourglass. But time can take the form of a gift, too. One person might view a cancelled appointment as a source of stress while another could see it as this rare gift of time that has dropped in his lap. Maybe that hour will be your opportunity to finally clean or arrange or inventory something that you've been neglecting. Maybe that snowstorm will be your wonderful day to stay at home and play with your kids. Make the most of these "gifts of time" whenever they present themselves.

Stress: Time Management's Worst Enemy

Stress, which we all experience to some degree or another, can make us run around like chickens without heads. We will talk about stress in more depth elsewhere in this book, but it is important to think about its impact on time management.

◉ Stress is the enemy of time management. It eats up time. You have to find ways to counter the stress so that you can stay with your time management system. For some people, that's deep breathing. For others it's yoga or listening to music. Do whatever works.

◎ When my stress level goes off the charts, I give myself a time-out. I do something that feels good. I work near a park, so a walk on a nice day is always a good choice. If the weather's not cooperating, I might go out for coffee or call a friend. Anything that gets me out of the stress.

◎ Having managed many people over the course of many years, I now understand that a lot of stress comes as a result of people not having good problem-solving skills. I've watched people walk around, eating themselves up about some unsolved problem, when they could just as well have figured things out with a little deductive reasoning and logic.

◎ Stress is a killer. It makes you work overtime by taxing your body, leaving you too worried to eat, sleep, or enjoy life. You've got to fight that kind of drain by making up a schedule of all your daily needs and keeping to it. Doing this gives you a strong sense of when you should be eating, resting, sleeping, and so on.

◎ You want to know how I beat stress? By giving myself goodies. Whenever I've come through a rough patch where I'm running myself ragged,

I reward myself with a special treat. Maybe it's a fruit smoothie, maybe it's a half-hour in a bubble bath, maybe it's a nap.

◎ I know people who pop tranquilizers like breath mints. I'm not knocking medication—as long as it's under strict doctor's orders—but a great free medicine with absolutely no bad side effects is exercise. A good workout is the best stress-buster in the world.

Learning to Say "No"

Learning to say "no" is a critical step in the overall scheme of saving time. Without the ability to say no, you will be chronically overloaded, often to the point of desperation. Some people have an especially hard time with the "N" word. Practicing in front of a mirror can be a helpful way to overcome this problem. Role play this for instance:

Boss: Jane, we need you to stay late tonight. Abby's got a doctor's appointment.

You: Sorry, Paul. I wish I could help you, but I've got to get home.

Boss: Can't you be a little flexible?

> You: Paul, remember I told you about my daughter's piano recital tonight?
>
> Boss: Oh yeah. You're right. Sorry. I'll ask Ivan.
>
> Saying "no" may take a lot of practice, depending on how out-of-the-habit you've gotten. But don't give up. You can do it!

There is Nothing Like a List

You may not think of yourself as a "list" sort of person, but the fact is that few of us can survive without them. A to-do list is the plumb line that keeps our days level and sane. Whether you use a pocket calendar, an electronic organizer, a stick-it pad, or ballpoint pen on the palm of your hand, don't leave home without it! You'll want a daily to-do list for sure, and may also find a weekly or even monthly to-do list beneficial.

◉ I've made the time I spend with my to-do list into a sacred daily routine. I used to review my list first thing in the morning—over coffee— and that was okay, but lately, I've been doing it before I go to bed at night and I like that even better. I know no one is going to disturb me and so I have 10 or 15 minutes to look over my list, and think in a peaceful and calm way about the day that's coming up.

◎ I have one rule I never break: I keep my to-do list to one page. If it's more than one page, that means there's too much to do on my to-do list!

◎ This may seem obvious, but I think prioritizing is central to making your to-do list. Decide what is the most important thing that you have to do and put that at the top of your list. In other words, Job Review with Boss goes at the top of the list and Cleaning the Grout around the Bathtub goes at the bottom, or off the list altogether.

◎ I think to-do lists are as individualized as fingerprints. I'm sure everybody's looks different. Mine has two columns. One says Hard, the other says Easy. If I know I have some easy stretches ahead of me, I can deal with the hard parts.

◎ One of the things I keep in mind when I organize my to-do list is what times of day I have the most energy. I know, for instance, that when four o'clock in the afternoon rolls around, I'm good for nothing. That's when I pencil in "coffee break." At eleven in the morning, however, I'm full of beans so I put down some high-energy task in that time slot.

- It's really important to understand that your to-do list is not set in stone or written in indelible ink. You can change things or shuffle them around. Think of your list as a guideline, that's all. It's not meant to intimidate, frustrate, or annihilate you!

- It's only in the last year or so that I've started keeping a weekly to-do list. When I was starting out, I didn't feel like I could cope with anything more than one day at a time, so all I did was a daily to-do list. But now that I've been with the same salon for close to five years, I feel more expansive. I can bite off bigger chunks of time and try to bring some perspective to them. So I not only look at the daily list, but I make a weekly to-do list and take on bigger projects that way Next step is the monthly list!

- The same way that I prioritize my daily to-do list is how I prioritize my weekly list. For example, I tell myself that I can only watch three hours of television a week, no matter what. I just don't have time for more and it turns my brain to jelly. So I pick my programs carefully.

- Everybody's got his own method but my "sanity secret" is to schedule in at least one block of free time a day. No matter how jam-packed a day I'm anticipating, I factor in free time. That way, I've got protection in case something unexpected comes up like car trouble, baby-sitting trouble, or whatever. And something unexpected always comes up!

◎ Not only are to-do lists valuable, but now that I use a real organizer, I see how many other great aids there are at my disposal. My organizer, for instance, has an insert that helps me keep track of expenses and my girlfriend uses one of those electronic organizers that practically runs her life!

◎ I always carry a pen and pad with me wherever I go. You never know when a good idea might strike. Never depend on your ability to remember it later. That's one of life's great lies.

◎ Good communication may be the best time-saver of all. Spend the extra time up front to find out what the client really wants so you don't have to spend twice as much time redoing what you did. Asking the right questions will save you the most time.

The Lost and Found of Time

If you keep close tabs on how you use your time over the course of a few weeks, chances are you'll be appalled by how much of it slips through your fingers. All of us can save hours a week by becoming aware of certain little short-cuts and fast ones we can pull on old Father Time.

At Work

Obviously, there are innumerable ways that people save time around the salon. Most of it is very individualized and has to do with personal style. One stylist we spoke with, however, offered an excellent distillation of time-saving efficiency methods that he calls "The Five Ps: Prior Planning Prevents Poor Performance."

1. Get to work early. Prepare yourself for the day. Have all your tools ready, as well as all the products that you will need in the salon, and make sure that the back bar is stocked. You don't want to have to stop your work to take care of these details.

2. Check your appointment book the night before. Make sure that your schedule maximizes your efficiency. How about doing a haircut while another client's perm is processing? Could you blow-style one client while doing a color treatment on another?

3. Always keep the salon as neat as you can. Clean while you go. Clutter only slows you down. Think of all the valuable time you waste looking for your shears.

4. Have the next client ready when you finish the one you're working on. Make sure that she is in a smock and ready to go.

5. Don't allow your clients to make you run behind. Sometimes it cannot be avoided—certain chemical services are unpredictable and may take longer such as color—but always factor in "late" time when you're scheduling so that you can run a little late on one appointment and not endanger the next one. Then rebook the tardy client.

Away from Work

There's no end to the ways you can save time when you start paying attention to your use of it. The following tips will give you some ideas of ways to own your time again in all the many areas of your life.

Shopping and Cooking

◉ Cooking can eat up much too much time, but you don't have to let it. You can still be considered a really good cook just using a repertoire of meals that you can cook in 30 minutes or less. You'll find all kinds of cookbooks out there that specialize in good, fast cooking.

◉ Double quantities when cooking whenever you can. If you freeze away the extras, you'll have two or three meals for the "time price" of one.

◉ I keep a shopping list with a pencil on a string on the refrigerator door. Whenever I use something up, I write it on the list. Then I go to the store with a friend or one of my kids, tear the list in half, and we meet back at the checkout, having done the job in half the time.

◎ My trick—when it comes to shopping—is to always shop in the same supermarket. Super-markets today are so huge that if you go to a new one where you're unfamiliar, it will take you three times as long. When I go to the same one all the time, I know exactly where the onions, light bulbs, paper towels, and cat food are.

Around the House

◎ I'm the President of the International I Hate Cleaning Society. The same way I prioritize my to-do list is how I prioritize my housecleaning. I figure out what needs to be done on a daily basis (picking up dirty clothes off the floor), on a weekly basis (cleaning the bathrooms, throw-ing out garbage, a little light vacuuming), what needs to be done monthly (I don't know, chang-ing the linen?), and yearly (Turning the mat-tress? Washing the windows? Yeah, right!).

◎ I keep cheap hand vacuums on every level of the house. I hardly ever take out the regular vacuum except maybe if company is coming.

◎ In our house, everyone has a cubby. That's where coats, hats, gloves, and shoes go. As for me, I always keep my keys and wallet in the same place. I used to be less careful about that, and I'd spend hours every week looking for things and dealing with extra stress that I needed like a hole in the head.

◎ One of the things that used to eat up a lot of my time was looking for stuff. Scissors, scotch tape, screwdrivers; everyday stuff like that. Then I had this brainstorm. I could buy four screwdrivers at $.99 apiece and I could keep them in strategic parts of the house. Same for scissors, tape, and all those other little things you're always misplacing. It's great!

Laundry

◎ If you have kids, the rule is white socks only! I don't want to hear any whining about how they have to have polka dots or little teddy bears on their socks. Everyone wears white and all things are equal.

◎ Consider a sleeping bag for your kids' beds instead of linen. They'll be just as happy, laundering will be easier, and there are no beds to make up.

Home Maintenance

◎ Silhouette your tools on a pegboard so you'll know just where everything goes.

◎ If you're always in a panic looking for warranties and appliance manuals and stuff like that, do what I did. Get a three-ring binder, punch holes in those important papers, and keep them all together where you will always know where to find them.

◉ It's a little thing but it makes me crazy: the amount of time it takes to untangle stuff like electric cords, Christmas tree lights, garden hoses, and whatever else has the capacity to get tangled. Now I put everything like that on reels and it saves me a lot of grief.

Travel

◉ I do a lot of shows, which means I travel all the time. I keep a master list of everything I need to take with me: my makeup, shampoo, alarm clock, and pharmaceuticals. Before I leave the house on any trip, I check off on my master list and I almost never get caught without the things I need.

◉ I like to keep an extra cosmetic bag packed just for travel so it's always ready to go.

◉ If I can, I get foreign currency ahead of time.

Miscellaneous Time Savers

◉ I try to cut down on all unnecessary trips. For instance, if I'm out shopping and my gas tank is still half full, I'll fill it anyway so I won't have to make a special trip at some other point just to get gas.

- The Internet has changed my life! I take advantage of all kinds of online services like automatic banking, shopping, and whatever.

- I relaxed my standards. In the past, if I wanted to have friends over, I'd feel that I'd have to make a beautiful dinner. Well, you can imagine how many friends I had to dinner, given my schedule and that mind-set. Now when I have friends over, everyone brings a dish. It's fun and it's easy.

- I make all my short calls to arrange appointments early in the day. That gives me something to cross off my to-do list which is a great way to start the day!

- Make the best use of your commute. If you're in walking distance of work, walk the walk and make this into your exercise time. If you're sitting on a bus or a subway, you might take this time to learn a new skill or you might further organize your to-do list or catch up on some much-needed sleep. If you're driving, check out books on tape. You can learn so much about so many different things while you're stuck in traffic.

- If the idea of hiring help makes sense and is within your budget, give this option careful consideration. Many of us are relentless "do-it-yourselfers" and feel that it is too much of a luxury or a cop-out to hire someone to clean our house, fix our leaky faucets, or change a pane of broken glass. It is all well and good to do these things yourself, but there are only so many hours in the day. If you can charge $50 for an hour of your time servicing a client, it may make sense to hire a housecleaner who charges $25 an hour for work.

◎ Buy a telephone answering machine if you don't already have one. That way, you can monitor incoming calls and decide when and if you want to take them. For instance, if you come home and you need an hour to be by yourself or with your family, you can get back to the caller at some other point. Another option is to consider getting rid of your answering machine. That way, you'll never have to return a call!

◎ I like to take advantage of down time. For me, it begins first thing in the morning. I set my alarm a half-hour before I actually have to get up and then luxuriate in bed before I have to confront another hectic day ahead of me.

◎ Think about what you have to do on a given day and bring a geographical perspective to it. In other words, if you have three errands in the north part of town, two in the south, and one in the east, make sure you plot it all out in a way that makes sense rather than retracing your steps.

◎ If you have kids, *carpool, carpool, carpool*! It's insane to live any other way.

Beating the Morning Madness

Mornings are the hardest for many people, particularly if you live in a house with many people (or any people other than you!). Here are some ways that your peers have found to make the mornings go smoother:

◎ Teach your family to pack their school bags, briefcases, the baby's diaper bag, and whatever else is needed for the day the night before and put them by the door.

◎ Lay out your work clothing the night before. If you're *really* good, you might want to use Sunday night to arrange your work wardrobe for the week. It takes a load off to know that you have five days of clean, ironed clothing ahead of you.

◎ Keep a chalkboard, a dry-erase board, or a pencil and pad by the door for any last-minute messages or notes.

◎ A bowl of coins goes a long way toward commutes, tolls, school lunches, money for a newspaper, and so forth. Make a routine of emptying your pockets into the bowl at night.

◎ Either you or your children can pack school lunches the night before and stick them in the fridge.

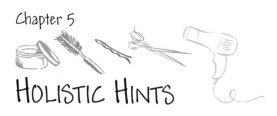

Chapter 5

HOLISTIC HINTS

magine yourself as an athlete with a big sports event coming up or an actor looking toward a major theatrical opening. You would be doing everything in your power to prepare yourself physically and mentally for your big day, wouldn't you? Well, as a cosmetologist, you know that *every* day in this field is a big day. If business is good, you should expect to be heavily booked. Countless demands will be made on you and there is always the stressful potential for making mistakes. There is a lot at stake and you have to perform. So, like that athlete or actor, you need to keep yourself in tip-top mental and physical condition. You have to look at The Whole You.

The idea of "wholeness" is at the heart of the word holistic, which means to emphasize the organic or functional relation between the parts and the whole of something. If we take a holistic approach to our lives, we are emphasizing ourselves as whole persons, not as a set of isolated functions.

In looking holistically at ourselves, we take into account mind, body, spirit, and how all of these interact and impact on each other. To neglect one part will, over time, negatively affect another part. In this chapter, we will be looking at ways in which your fellow cosmetologists hold it all together and stay healthy and whole.

You Are What You Eat

So goes the famous old saying, and there's a great deal of truth to it. What we put into our bodies has a great deal of bearing on how well we function. Think about your nutrition and take note of what your fellow cosmetologists have to say on the subject.

◉ Water, water everywhere! That's the key. Our bodies are 60 percent to 70 percent water, so you have to replenish whatever you lose. The more you hydrate, the better you'll feel and function. Drink at least eight 8-ounce glasses a day. (Don't overdo, however, and drink gallons. That can cause problems, too). I always take a large container of spring water to work with me. I keep it close by and I drink *before* I get thirsty. Keep in mind, too, that certain substances, like the caffeine in tea and coffee, can act as diuretics, causing water to leave your body. Don't depend on those beverages to hydrate you.

◎ I always pay attention to my diet to make sure that I've got a lot of variety. That way, I figure I'm covering my bases. If I eat dairy, grains, fruits, veggies, and a little chicken or fish, then I can feel pretty confident that I'm getting what I need. This means that I never go on diets where I'm mostly eating grapefruits or cabbage soup or steak or what have you.

◎ I believe in whole foods. Not everything I eat is organic, although I do try to eat organic when possible. But even when the foods are not organic, I still try to pick those that have the least processing. That means real cheese and not cheese food. Rolled oats instead of some sugar-packed cereal. Even a piece of semisweet chocolate if I have a sugar craving over some candy bar that's stuffed with marshmallow-nougat-brittle and that may have all kinds of artificial ingredients in it. When it comes to food, the less tampering the better.

◎ You want to hear a revolutionary concept? Don't eat when you're not hungry. Most of the time you're doing that, you're just trying to alleviate stress, which can be better dealt with by a few minutes of deep breathing or maybe a walk outside. You'd be amazed how much easier it is to keep your weight under control when you pay attention to your stomach hunger instead of your mouth hunger.

- My mother used to tell me to chew each bite of food 50 times. I couldn't stand it when she said that, but there is a lot of sense to it. As an adult, I find that if I eat slowly and chew my food thoroughly, I eat a lot less and I have a lot less stomach distress.

- Watch your portions. Americans are known throughout the world for eating totally excessive amounts of food. The idea of "doubling" it or ordering a 64-oz. soda is unheard of in most parts of the globe and should be unheard of here, too.

- I always bring my lunch from home. Even if I'm going out with a friend, I'd rather brown bag it with some good healthy food and take it to the park than wind up in some overpriced restaurant that's serving food of a quality I can't be sure. And don't even get me started on fast food! I see some of my coworkers eating at those places every day and I just want to say, "Don't you have a kitchen at home?"

- I try to avoid fads in foods. For instance, suddenly fat became a dirty word. I come from an

Italian family, and the idea of going without fats—cheese, olive oil, nuts—is unimaginable. Of course, now all the experts are praising "the Mediterranean diet," where fats like olive oil and nuts are shown to have enormous benefits. Fat is delicious and satisfying, and a little bit will sate your hunger. When we cut down on fat, we bulk up on carbohydrates, which, for most people, means highly refined foods like sugar, pastas, and white breads. Then you really have to start worrying about your weight.

◎ Get into the habit of reading labels. Find out what fat content works for your diet, what kind of fat is in a product (for instance, a label will tell you if a product has an unhealthy fat like partially hydrogenated coconut or palm kernel oils), how much sodium you should be having, any calcium benefits, and so on.

◎ People get very worried about their protein intake. Don't worry so much. You don't have to eat meat, fish, or chicken for protein. Think about beans and nuts, tofu, or maybe a protein supplement added to a smoothie or a shake. That's what I do. Every day, I put a full measure of protein powder in a blender with some orange juice and a frozen banana, and I don't have to worry about my daily protein intake at all.

◎ You want to know my secret to eating healthy? Make a nice meal out of every meal you have.

For breakfast, I always make sure there's some beautiful fruit on the plate. For lunch, I often have a thermos of hot soup and a wrap. For dinner, even if I'm by myself, I put down a placemat, pour myself a glass of wine, and eat a leisurely and relaxing meal. I think grabbing your food and gulping it down on the run is the worst thing you can do for yourself.

◉ Is there anyone left in the world who doesn't understand the importance of fiber? That means fruits, vegetables, legumes, and whole-grain breads and cereals. Better do it now, folks, or you'll be paying for it later.

Personal Hygiene

As a cosmetologist, it is important for you to always keep in mind that you are in the image business. People come to see you so that they can look good. If you don't look good, they will draw the conclusion that you can't make them look good. Looking good always starts with good personal hygiene. Most of the issues around personal hygiene are obvious and we will not insult your intelligence by even bringing them up here. As a working adult out in the world, surely you understand the importance of toothbrushes and deodorants. Instead, we will touch on a few hints that your fellow cosmetologists feel are useful for everyone to know and to incorporate into their lifestyles.

◎ We cosmetologists are in a people profession. We get very close to others throughout the day. To me, that means no garlic on the pizza. Seriously. I love garlic on pizza, but I'm not going to lose a client because of it. And believe me, you do lose clients over things like bad breath.

◎ The three most important words in your life? *Wash your hands!* Making this simple and free practice a religion will save you and your clients an enormous amount of grief.

◎ It seems as if I shouldn't have to tell other cosmetologists about the need to moisturize, but it's too important a hygiene issue to go unmentioned. Skin dries out so quickly, especially under conditions like central heating or air-conditioning, exposure to the sun, and what have you. Find a moisturizer you like and live with it. Carry it on your person. Use it on your face and your hands throughout the day. An ounce of prevention is worth pounds of cure!

◎ Everything about you is going to be an advertisement to your clients. That means your hair and certainly your nails. Ragged, dirty nails are going to make clients flee from you in droves. Why should they place their trust in someone who doesn't adhere to the standard they're aiming for?

◉ Say *au revoir* to perfume, if you're still wearing it. Perfume has its rightful place in the world, but the workplace is not its rightful place. A great many people are allergic to fragrances, and more and more salons are instituting a no-fragrance policy. If you feel you have to use fragrance, keep it as light as you can. A citrusy toilet water, for instance, but never some heavy, musky scent!

Personal Grooming and Style

Many salon owners and managers consider appearance, personality, and poise to be just as important for success as technical knowledge and skills. So the question is: how are you doing in the grooming department?

◉ I am personally quite surprised and sometimes appalled by the way some of my coworkers, particularly the younger ones, maintain—or should I say, fail to maintain—their wardrobes. Clothing is stained or ripped. Buttons are missing. Sweaters are so pilled as to be unsightly. Whites are yellowed. Don't they understand the first thing they need to do to keep themselves looking fresh?

- Sometimes, I think certain people would benefit from taking an adult ed course in laundry. Really, it's as if they never got the basics down. When I used to go to a laundromat, I'd watch people stuffing things into the washer. Well, if you want to get clothes clean, you need to give them room to move around. Also, the idea of separating lights from darks seems to elude certain people. To throw a white blouse in with a black sweatshirt . . . go figure.

- Clothing may look clean, but when you're working close to a client—and cosmetology is one of the most intimate professions—you can't just *look* clean. You have to *smell* clean. I hang my clothes out to dry in the sun. Nothing makes clothes smell cleaner than that.

- Ever hear of an iron? I manage a salon, and I've got people coming in to work wearing shirts and blouses that look like they were retrieved from the bottom of the laundry hamper. Come on, folks. Ironing is something you can do while you watch television. It's not so terrible!

- My pet peeve is crummy-looking shoes. Some people will really put themselves together and look just fine until you get down to their feet. Shoes need to be cleaned, like any other part of your wardrobe, and a good polish helps, too. Downtrodden heels aren't the world's best look either. I know it's hard to find a shoemaker these days, but that doesn't mean that you can get away with shoes that look like junk.

◎ Fact of life: some people's feet don't smell so good. That's probably because they perspire a lot, which is healthy and fine, and is usually addressed by civilized people with underarm deodorant. But people perspire through the soles of their feet as well, you know, particularly when you're on your feet all day long, walking the equivalent of I don't know how many miles. So I always keep a natural foot powder on hand and I use it liberally during the day. I also always have at least two pairs of good work shoes that I alternate from one day to the next, so that one pair can air out while I'm wearing the other pair.

◎ My advice for developing a good professional wardrobe is to buy more than one of something you really love. This might sound like an extravagance, and maybe your budget really can't handle buying in multiples, but over the long run, when you have a shirt or a sweater that gets an A+ on appearance, comfort, and durability, then it makes great economic sense to buy more than one. Chances are, you'll buy two or three things like it to try to match up to the much-loved one when it kicks the bucket, and you'll never be as happy.

◎ This may seem incredibly obvious, but the best way to get a good wardrobe for work (or play) is to buy on sale. I don't mean discount shopping, which, to me, takes a whole lot of time and can be very hit and miss. I mean buying at the end of the season. If you go into any department store or chain in February to buy winter clothes for next year, you'll pay literally about a third of what you'll pay in October for these same winter clothes. And if you buy classic styles, you won't have to worry about what's going to be in or out next year. You can pay top dollar if you want to accessorize when the new fashions come out, but buy your staples when they're giving them away.

◉ As a manager, I try to kindly, gently, and subtly suggest to some of the youngsters who come to work here that they don't have to show up looking like a Christmas tree. You know what I mean? Some of them wear so much jewelry and try for so much flash. It's a lot to keep up and can be very distracting. I would tell a young stylist that it's a good idea to try to have your hair, your makeup, and your clothing blend in with the surroundings of your salon. Look around the salon. If everyone is very minimalist, don't come in looking flashy. It's only common sense.

◉ It gets into a touchy area when you start trying to control a person's appearance. Appearance is an expression of who that person is, and you don't want to appear to be squelching that.

That said, however, I feel as a manager that I have to draw a line at certain places. Clothing that is exhibitionist just won't fly with our clientele, so I keep a smock on hand for any stylist who comes in looking like she's dressed for a hot night.

◎ As a manager, I think there's a lot to be said for uniforms. I love working in a salon where everyone is wearing the same crisp, clean, and smartly-cut outfit. It feels very professional and easy to me.

◎ Uniforms can be a great solution for the salon, but even if you're working in a salon with a no-uniform policy, you might want to create a uniform of your own. In other words, keep your wardrobe very simple, classic, and easy, and you'll convey a sense of style and utility that others will want to copy. I think good choices for such a uniform are simple: A-line skirts in muted colors with a white or black silk T-shirt, for instance. For a guy, it might be a white shirt, a tie, and clean, tailored khakis. These uniforms project just the kind of professional appearance and attitude that may allow you to charge more for your services.

◎ It's one of those weird quirks of human nature, but did you ever notice how someone who's a builder can have the most run-down home? I've known hairdressers like that. They cut other people's hair all day long and they allow their own hair to get long and ratty or faded. Bad idea!

◎ One little (well, maybe not so little) thing that drives me crazy: I see some of the other girls in the salon sharing makeup. That is such a bad thing to do! Makeup is a breeding ground for bacteria and should never be shared with anyone else. Sharing can lead to conjunctivitis, sties, herpes, and don't ask! I keep makeup for six months and then get rid of it. I start in with new, fresh makeup that's just for me.

Healthy Body, Healthy Mind

Moving on from the externals of one's appearance, let's have a look at how other cosmetologists focus in on ways to protect and sustain the inner person. We'll start once again with the issue of stress, which is a big concern for all people in the world today (stress is so present in our lives that the World Health Organization classified it as an epidemic in a 1992 United Nations Report labeled *Job Stress: The 20th Century Disease*) but is particularly prevalent in the field of cosmetology.

◎ Why is this field so stressful? Because you have to perform for clients and for your boss. You have to be technically proficient and you have to be able to get along with people. You have to be able to organize your time and be self-promoting yet discreet. You have to be able to sell somebody something, which for some people is one of the most stressful aspects of the field. Throw into all this the fact that you are dealing with an incredibly wide and unpredictable range of personalities, and the fact that you're on your feet all day. And what do you get? Stress!

◎ Stress can come out of the interpersonal relationships that are going on in the salon, but obviously it can also come out of the interpersonal relationships that you have outside of the salon. If you're having problems with your partner, or with your kids or parents or a friend, you're going to have stress, and meeting the demands of a stressful job is not going to be easy. You can also have stress from factors that have nothing to do with your interrelationships with other people. For instance, you might be having a bad reaction to some substance you're using at work, and this could be causing you and your body a great deal of stress.

◎ I have coworkers who deal with stress by taking anti-anxiety drugs, and I'm certainly not knocking that if it's what you need (as long as you're carefully following doctor's orders, that is). Some of my coworkers, however, deal with stress by getting bombed after work or by cutting out of the salon every hour for a smoke. I am knocking those antistress responses. Why? Because they cause you and your body to suffer a lot more stress over the long run. To me, the way to deal with stress is by finding even a small amount of time every day to go inside of yourself and to connect with your spiritual side. Whether you do that by meditation, prayer, yoga, a walk in the woods or in the park, or simply by deep breathing is up to you. But you've got to do it.

- I think deep breathing is the best stress reliever there is. It calms yet energizes simultaneously. It can also lower blood pressure. Now, you're going to ask me how you can breathe deeply when you're feeling stressed and can't get a deep breath, right? Good question. It's something you learn how to do. Go to a yoga class and find out.

- I do deep breathing with a twist. When I'm stressed, I tell myself to breathe in the good as I'm breathing in and breathe out the bad as I'm breathing out. You'd be amazed how forceful an antistress action this is. And you can do it anywhere. I've been known to run into a toilet stall and do it when I have to.

- My cure for stress is sleep. I know a lot of people can't sleep when they're stressed, but for me it's the opposite. I make a point of getting into bed before 10 PM with some Celtic music on and a lavender candle burning, and I'm good for eight hours.

◎ Laughing helps. When I'm stressed out, I turn off the news on the car radio and I put on my tapes instead. When I laugh, I can feel the stress leaving my body. Try it, you'll see.

◎ If you're under a lot of stress (and who isn't these days?), make sure you get your B vitamins. Calcium, too. Stay away from foods that put a lot of stress on your body like colas, fried foods, chips, junk food, white sugar, all that stuff. Eating a lot of raw foods is beneficial in a stress situation.

◎ Exercise, ladies and gentlemen. Plenty of it. And it doesn't have to be exercise that you don't enjoy in order for it to be good for you. In fact, it shouldn't be exercise you don't enjoy. Tennis, soccer, inline skating, aerobic dancing are all great. Just make sure the exercise is regular.

◎ I've got a secret weapon against stress: vacations! Seriously, a lot of us forget to take them, particularly if we're working for ourselves. The therapeutic effect of a vacation can be enormous. Even a day off when you're feeling really stressed out can make a world of difference. Spend the day bicycling or pack a picnic and head for the beach. You'll feel like a new person.

◎ For me, it's hobbies. My friends think I'm crazy but I like to build birdhouses. I've made about 400 of them so far. I'm running out of people to give them to.

◎ I got better at coping with stress once I weaned myself from caffeine. It's a personal decision, but if you're suffering from stress, you might want to experiment with substituting a nice herbal tea for some of that coffee you've been chugging. Some herbs, which you'll find in teas, have natural stress-relieving properties such as Chamomile, rose hips, and ginseng. Check them out.

 Physical Presentation

Another important aspect of professional image is what is called physical presentation. To a large degree, your physical presentation is made up of your posture, walk, and movements. Your physical presentation enhances or detracts from your attractiveness, and is also an important part of your well-being. Unhealthy or defective body postures can cause a number of musculoskeletal problems, particularly when these postures become habit. Here are some ideas from your colleagues about how to keep your body healthy and functioning at peak level in the workplace.

◎ When I started on my first job, I was taken under the wing by another stylist, a wonderful woman who went on to become a real mentor to me. One of the first things she did was to give me a mini-course in posture. It has kept me in good shape all the years since. Basically, she gave me a set of rules that I have always followed, and it goes like this: Head up and chin level with the floor; neck elongated and balanced directly above the shoulders; chest out and up; shoulders level, spine straight; abdomen flat; hips level horizontally; and knees slightly flexed and positioned over the feet. This is something you've got to learn how to do, and learning it is not easy, but once you've got it down, it will protect you for your whole career.

◎ Just as important as your standing posture is your sitting posture. The one thing I always tell the people who work for me is slide your rear to the rear. It takes discipline to do that. Many of us sprawl in our chairs. But if you tuck your tush into the back of the chair, your body will be grateful.

◎ I travel around the country as an educator and I see manicurists all the time who are sitting on a little bit of their stool. I say to them, "It's designed for your entire bottom, dear." Check out what I'm talking about and you'll see the difference.

- When you're sitting, keep your back straight and the soles of your feet on the floor. Don't cross your legs or your feet at the ankle. Your soles on the floor give you support.

- You know what makes me laugh? And then makes me shake my head with pity? Stylists working in high heels! Are they crazy or what? Whether the heels are chunky or narrow doesn't matter: both apply pressure to the knees. They also throw off your center of gravity, and leave you open to a host of problems like back pain and arthritis. Leave them in the closet for those special occasions only.

- Get yourself a good pair of shoes. No, get yourself at least two good pairs of shoes. Something nice and wide and low-heeled that will absorb shock and give your toes the room they need. Don't leave home without them!

- If your salon is not carpeted, treat yourself to a cushioned mat for your station. It'll go a long way toward beating fatigue.

- In the course of a day, you're probably going to walk the equivalent of ten miles, so pamper your feet when you get home at night. Massage them with some oil after showering, and then thoroughly dry them, especially between the toes, and apply an antiseptic foot lotion or a natural foot powder. Regular pedicures are worth every penny toward keeping your feet in good condition.

◎ All of us working in this field are very susceptible to cumulative trauma disorder (CTDS). We have to stand all day and hold our bodies in unnatural positions for long periods of time, which means we're contracting our muscles. This can lead to problems of the hands, wrists, shoulders, neck, back, feet, and legs. Prevention is the key here. You've got to fit your work to your body, not your body to your work.

◎ There are certain ergonomic measures we must all be aware of. One of them is to adjust the height of your chair with each client, and to swivel the chair as much as you need to so you don't overextend your reach.

◎ People lapse into bad habits, even those of us with good techniques. What I do is to have another stylist watch me now and then to make sure I'm not doing anything I shouldn't be doing. I ask them to evaluate my technique. They might tell me that I'm not keeping my wrists as straight as they should be, for instance, and then I'll make corrections.

◎ Here's a short and sweet one. Hold your blow-dryer sideways so you don't have to raise your arms above shoulder level any more than you have to.

◉ Sharp shears make a big difference. Sharp, well-balanced, and well-lubricated shears mean you don't have to work as hard to cut hair.

◉ Keep your elbows as close to your sides as possible.

◉ I always try to keep my back straight, and I always, always, always bend at the hips or knees instead of at the waist.

◉ Study the flamingo. They stand for long periods of time by resting on one foot. If you're standing for a long time, try placing one foot on a stool for a while. You'll see the difference.

◉ When you're giving a manicure, always have your client extend her hand across the table to you, not the other way around. If you're extending your hands and arms all day to your clients, you'll wear yourself out in no time.

◉ A lot of ergonomic issues are matters that you can address personally, but then you have to understand that there are other ergonomic issues that need to be dealt with institutionally. For instance, work stations need to have ample space between them so that your movement is not restricted. Cabinets should be within easy reach. Freestanding shampoo bowls allow shampooing to be done from behind instead of from the side, where your body is twisted sideways, which can cause or aggravate back problems. Before you take a job with a salon, check out these issues. If you are working in a salon where there are such issues, you and your coworkers might want to meet with management to see about remedying the problems.

◉ If you work in an environment that has any physical discomfort built into it, as most of us do, try to counter the problem by including regular stretching intervals in your schedule to break up the repetitiveness of the motions you use.

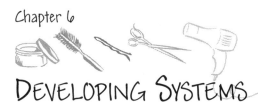

Chapter 6

DEVELOPING SYSTEMS

As a cosmetologist, no matter where you are—if you have a job in a salon or if you are working for yourself—there is a great deal for which you have to personally take responsibility. Even if you are working in a national chain of salons and think that everything is all laid out for you, this is not really the case. A certain sense of autonomy and independence will help you grow in your profession, regardless of your situation, and will lead you toward greater career success.

You will find that you work best when you create powerful systems for yourself. For example, you will want to create the most efficient work area possible. You will have to organize your files and paperwork. You will want to find ways of standing and sitting that will treat your body well, and preserve it for the length of your career. You'll need to take care of your skin, which is constantly exposed to moisture and chemicals.

In this chapter, we will have a look at ways that your fellow cosmetologists have created high-functioning systems for themselves in the areas we've mentioned above.

 ## The Work Area

This is your home base, and you need to make it is as organized and sanitary as possible.

- As far as product is concerned, I like to keep the minimum at the station. That means one spray, one water bottle, and a gel. Of course, you'll keep your combs in the proper disinfectant as well

- I buy those plastic organizers you find in household stores that people use in their kitchen drawers, and I use them to organize my combs, shears, and any other loose items that need to be contained.

- After each client, I put my blow-dryer on cold and use it to blow away the hair from my station and surrounding area, including the styling chair, which makes it easier for the assistants to sweep up. I also clean out my station cabinet, top, and drawers the same way. It's like a leaf blower: fast!

- Make sure that your floors are swept clean after each service. Nothing makes a worse impression on an incoming client than having to look at the debris of the client you served before.

- Need I point out that food has no place at your work area? In our salon, we used to call one of the stylists "Pizza Man" because he always had a slice at his station.

- Empty your waste receptacle more than less. Believe me, no one wants to look at an overflowing waste basket.

- Make sure to close all containers after you've used them. Some people rush around and leave them open until the end of a service. This opens them up to contamination and does not give a professional appearance.

- I check every container on my counter at the end of the day to wipe off any drips or whatever. That's just basic daily routine for me because I don't want my clients to see a lot of icky-sticky-yucky-looking jars and whatnot on my counter.

- I've worked in places where basic disinfection is not followed, and believe me, that's scary.

Before and after each client, you must use an EPA-registered, hospital-grade disinfectant on your work surface, and you've got to leave it on for the full amount of time prescribed by the manufacturers' directions. All surfaces of the work area have to be disinfected, which means knobs, handles, and so forth. If this isn't basic protocol in your salon, find out why or look for another job.

◉ In our salon, we keep a rolling cart on the floor that holds one of every product we either use or retail. This helps keeps your station clean and clear. And it winds up being more cost-effective because you're not wasting lots of product.

◉ I'm known as The White Tornado in our salon, and I really get on people's nerves sometimes, but I don't care. There are certain standards that need to be met, and if they aren't met, you're opening yourself up to disaster. So anyone who comes into my salon has to listen to and learn Gloria's Golden Ten:

1. wash hands after using the rest room and between clients

2. use disposable drinking cups only

3. no food is permitted in any refrigerators that are used to store salon products

4. freshly-laundered towels are a must for each client

5. capes or coverings are never to touch a client's skin

6. no sharing of makeup, lipsticks, puffs, pencils, or brushes is allowed

7. use clean spatulas, not your fingers, to remove products from containers

8. no tools, hairpins, rollers, or combs are to be placed in the stylist's mouth for safekeeping

9. no pets or animals are *ever* invited into the salon with the exception of service dogs

10. client gowns and headbands must be laundered after each use.

Anyone cheating on any of the above is in big trouble!

For Your Safety

In addition to the above general rules of hygiene, stylists must follow rules of safety in a variety of specific situations.

◉ The first thing I tell my young stylists is to always wear gloves and safety glasses when mixing chemicals with waters. No shortcuts ever!

◉ Always add disinfectant to water, not water to disinfectant.

- Make sure to use tongs, gloves, or a draining basket to remove implements from disinfectant baths.

- I've seen people pour quats, phenols, formalin, and alcohol over their hands. It gives me the willies. It's really a pretty crazy thing to do because these substances can cause skin disease and can increase the risk of infection.

- Listen up, people: never, *ever*, place any disinfectant or any other product in an unlabeled container. This is one of the surest routes to disaster.

- Ultraviolet (UV) sanitizers are good for storage but don't think that they can be used for disinfecting salon implements.

- To prevent the spread of disease, all disposable supplies such as orangewood sticks, emery boards, cotton, gauze, and neck strips should be thrown away. Anything exposed to blood, including microdermabrasion debris, must be double-bagged and marked with a biohazard sticker, or marked and disposed of according to OSHA standards.

- A rule of thumb to be tattooed on your forehead or wherever you need to have it so that you remember it at all times is *disinfect or discard*. That's your choice.

Keeping Records

One of the most important aspects of a stylist's job is to keep scrupulous records of client services and any retail products that are sold to clients. You will not be able to trust your memory to recall exactly the color that Mrs. Jones wore to her daughter's wedding that she'd like to duplicate for her niece's wedding. Either a card file system or memorandum book kept in a central location will be necessary if you want to hold onto a growing clientele and satisfy their needs.

- The idea is to use the consultation card from the moment a new client calls the salon to make an appointment. Make sure that you, the receptionist, or whoever is booking the appointment has scheduled in 20 or 30 minutes of consultation time.

- You may have a new client who is not used to having consultations. You'll want to let her know that it is salon policy to gather certain information before you can begin the service and that it is important for her to arrive early enough to fill out a consultation card. In many salons, the receptionist calls to remind clients about their appointments the day before they are scheduled. This is a good time to remind the client that she will need to fill out a consultation card, which will probably take her five to ten minutes, with an additional ten minutes or so for the two of you to talk it over.

◎ All service records should include the name and address of the client, the date of each purchase or service, the amount charged, products used, and results obtained. Clients' preferences and tastes should also be noted

◎ It's particularly vital for colorists to keep accurate records. You might have a client who is absolutely thrilled with the magic you've worked and then, five weeks later, the client is back for more color work and you have no idea what formula you used. Oops! There goes the client.

◎ With color clients, I record all formulas, processing times, and any notes on porosity or other significant conditions. You know, when you're coloring, you'll often do one process on the ends and one on the roots. How are you going to remember things like that if you don't keep scrupulous records?

◎ I have a friend who's a great colorist but a lousy organizer. She had a client come in, and midway through the coloring, the client said, "Wait a minute! Last time I went from blonde to red." My friend looked at the blonde locks, looked at her notes, and realized she had forgotten to jot down the change. Unfortunately, the client didn't take the mix-up too well and went looking for another colorist.

- I keep a file box of 4 x 6 cards on which I carefully record everything I need to know about what I've done for a client such as formulas, processing times, porosity, and the like. If I have to do one process on the ends and another on the roots, that goes down on the card, too. A lot of work, you say? I wouldn't have it any other way!

- Not only do I keep notes of what I've actually done, but I write an ongoing narrative about how a service has turned out and what I think I could do better next time. I record my client's impressions and reservations, and any goals I'm working toward. All of that goes down on the card.

- Make sure other people can read your handwriting. If you happen to be out one day and a client needs to be serviced by another colorist, that colorist is going to have to read your notes.

- There are good software programs out there for storing and accessing all the color information and records you need.

- My incredible discovery for keeping records is a Palm Pilot. It stores many hundreds of records—believe me, I should have that many clients—and all I have to do is tap in whatever details I want and it all gets stored. The base color, the highlights . . . it's all there. My Palm also stores tons of other details about my clients like who referred them, their birthdays, what they do for a living, and so on. I love my Palm!

◉ Once you've finished the service, you'll hear from the client whether she's satisfied or not. Take a few more minutes to record these results on the record card. Make a note of anything you did that you might want to do again, as well as anything that you wish you could undo or, at the very least, never repeat. Also, make note of the condition of the client's hair after the service and jot down any retail products that you recommended for her purchase.

Ergonomics

Chances are you've heard the term ergonomics, but may not be so sure what it means exactly. Ergonomics is a response to the many work-related disorders that result when there is a mismatch between the physical capacity of workers and the demands of the job. Each year, hundreds of workers report musculoskeletal disorders including carpal tunnel syndrome, tendonitis, and back injuries. According to the definition provided by the Ergonomics Society, ergonomics is about fit: the fit between people, the things they do, the objects they use, and the environments in which they work, travel, and play. Ergonomics is of special concern to beauty professionals whose work takes a serious toll on their bodies.

◉ We cosmetologists expose our bodies to potential injury every day we're on the job. I know cosmetologists who are so physically exhausted that they can barely function. We have to stand all day long and hold our bodies in unnatural positions for extended periods of time, contracting our muscles in ways that may lead to chronic or cumulative trauma disorders. Some of these problems can become so serious that I know stylists who have actually had to leave the field.

◉ Okay, folks—here's the rule. *You fit your work to your body, not your body to your work.* You only get one body in this lifetime, so take great care of it.

◉ It is very important that you fit your work to your body, and not your body to your work. An awareness of your body posture and movements, coupled with better work habits, and proper tools and equipment, will greatly enhance your health and comfort.

◉ As a manager, I consider it to be a big part of my job to make sure that members of my staff are taking care of themselves and their physical needs. Look at the things we're doing all day long. So many of us, when we're cutting or holding a hair dryer or using the round brush, are constantly moving our wrists up and down instead of keeping them straight. We're using repetitive and forceful gripping motions, sometimes with shears or curling irons that are unbalanced or dull, or that don't fit well into our hands. The shoulder strain from holding our arms away from our bodies can get unbearable, and need I mention the neck and back strain from bending forward incorrectly or twisting our bodies to get closer to a client or to reach for something? All of these actions, over long periods of time, add up to a prescription for incapacitation. And the pity of it all is that so much of it can be avoided.

◎ To get into a better ergonomic place, you really should start by using your chair as it was meant to be used. That means adjusting its height with each client and swiveling it as often as necessary so you don't have to overextend your reach. I've watched stylists cutting hair who act like the chair is a stationary, straight-backed wooden chair. It's ridiculous!

◎ If you're finding the work exhausting, part of the problem may be that you're not letting the client do part of the work. The client should be tilting his head as you direct him so that you don't have to gyrate into positions to cut his hair.

◎ Our salon does a superb job of staying on top of ergonomic concerns. We have an assistant manager who has made ergonomics a special area of expertise. He's been to lots of seminars and classes and stuff, and he does regular reviews of how we cut hair from a strictly ergonomic point of view. He'll show us how to change our technique, for instance, to make sure that we're keeping our wrists as straight as possible.

◉ When I was a kid, my father taught me how to use a hammer and nails. "Let the hammer do the work," he told me, and it was great advice. That's what tools are designed for: to do the work. So make sure, for instance, that your shears are balanced, sharp, and lubricated. You'll see what a difference it makes in terms of your muscle strain.

◉ I always try to use my blow-dryer sideways. That way, I don't have to raise my arms above shoulder level that much.

◉ Elbows to the side, ladies and gentlemen. Try it. You'll feel the difference immediately.

◉ There are certain basic ergonomic rules that apply across the board in any and all fields that involve physical activity. Keeping your back straight is a biggie. Always bending at the knees and the hips, and never at the waist, is another.

◉ You know what's great for fatigue? Sitting down! Seriously, this simple measure is something that a lot of people seem to want to avoid. It's not a macho thing to do but because I have my hair-cutting stool and because I use it, I've got a lot more reserve of energy than a lot of those younger stylists. Even if I'm not sitting on the stool, I can stand and alternately rest a foot on the stool to relieve my fatigue.

◎ Don't even think about starting to cut hair in a salon without having a cushioned floor mat under your feet. If you're lucky, you're working in a carpeted salon where it won't be necessary, although even in those posh circumstances, you might want the added comfort of a foot mat. It does wonders!

◎ I wouldn't even think about taking any particular ergonomic measures before I got myself a good pair of shoes. That means low heels and lots of arch support. If you've got problems with flat feet or an overly high arch, you might want to go with orthopedic inserts. I see some of my coworkers spending long days in little sandals or whatever, and I think they're crazy. When I got out dancing, which I try to do about once a month because I love it, I wear my dancing shoes. But I'm not going to wear dancing shoes to work.

◎ I was exhausting myself physically but then I decided to cut back on my hours. I never work longer than five hours at a stretch now. I'm sorry, but if I didn't do that, I wouldn't be able to work at all.

- I get massages regularly and pedicures. My feet need to be in great shape. It's worth every penny.

- If you haven't discovered yoga yet, don't delay. Yoga moves can be done almost anywhere and they bring so much relief.

- Regular stretching is extremely beneficial to your body. Schedule a few minutes of stretching time in between each appointment.

Analyzing Your Ergonomic Environment

An ergonomically healthy situation is not only dependent on the measures you take to protect yourself, but is also a result of what the salon does to protect you. You should have an awareness of certain ergonomic standards, and if your salon is not meeting them, you may want to suggest changes. If you feel these suggestions would not be welcomed and if the situation is serious enough, you may have to consider looking elsewhere for employment. As favorable as certain aspects of your job may be, you will not be able to work at the job long if the ergonomic environment is unhealthy.

- Let's start with the air quality. Four to ten air changes per hour are recommended for public buildings. The air changes remove suspended particles such as hairspray, nail filings, and microscopic particles loosened when brushing the scalp. Hopefully, you have found yourself in a salon with an air purification system or an EPA-registered air cleaner/deodorizer spray that can remove these particles.

- Some salons try to cram as many chairs into a space as they can. This has the potential to make your life miserable. Work stations should have adequate space between them so that a stylist does not have to restrict her movements. You don't want to feel strait-jacketed when you're working.

- You should be looking for hydraulic chairs that adjust up and down by at least five inches. You should expect to have cabinets that don't require you to strain yourself to get what you need. And you really should have freestanding shampoo bowls that allow you to shampoo from behind the chair instead of from the side. The twisting involved in shampooing from the side can lead to back problems in no time.

- If you perform manicures, your table should have an armrest on which you can place your wrists, allowing you to keep the knuckles below the wrists as you work on the client's hands.

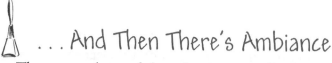

... And Then There's Ambiance

The atmosphere of the salon is generally determined by the management, but there are certain aspects of the ambiance that you might control or at least have input on. One is odors and the other is music.

Controlling and Eliminating Odors

◎ The odors from perms and color can be completely overwhelming, particularly to a lot of my male clients, so I think the odor problem is a big one. If you're in a smaller salon like I am, the costs of installing a venting system in the ceiling that vents outside is a fortune, even though that's clearly the best way to deal with the situation. We took a less expensive but worthwhile route, which was to buy a purification system. It's very quiet, and even though it doesn't zap the odor on contact, it keeps it from hanging around in the salon.

◎ I use scented candles. Not everybody loves them but most people do. I don't go for some heavy, perfumey scent, but instead use a nice clean lemony candle. Sometimes, at holiday time, I'll burn some cinnamon candles. If I'm expecting a male client, I might use a lavender candle. Men seem to like lavender for some reason.

◎ We put ceiling fans into our salon and they circulate the air, which cuts down a lot on odors.

Of course, I don't think there's an odor-free salon in the world, so don't expect one.

◎ Candles are good, but I prefer aromatherapy oils in special little electric burners or in rings on the lightbulbs. Of course, with a candle or any burner, you have to be very careful about stuff like hairspray. But you have to be careful in the salon generally, right?

◎ A great way to eliminate odors is to open the window! Some salons become so dependent on controlled environments that they don't realize there is fresh air outside that is absolutely free and better at countering odors than anything that man has invented.

Salon Music

A lot of battles have broken out in salons over the issue of what kind of music is going to be playing in the background. Here are how some individuals have solved the problem.

◎ We were having a lot of disputes in our salon on this issue. Everyone wanted something different, so we went out and got a CD changer that holds 24 CDs. Everyone brings in three favorite CDs; we collectively judged them all and picked, by democratic vote, the top 24. Now that's what's on the changer. Once a month, we change the whole thing by going through the same process. A little time-consuming maybe, but it beats all the energy that goes into the fights we used to have about music.

- After a lot of discussion, we agreed to listen only to a light rock station. It may not be everyone's favorite genre, but it's the one choice that everyone felt they could live with.

- We discovered something great: a satellite dish that has 100 channels with everything from rock to country to opera to jazz to Broadway and on and on. There are no storage issues, the price is low, nothing gets pilfered, and you can make changes as you want. Also, many people don't realize that they are supposed to pay fees for playing a radio station or CD in a public place. Satellite or cable are two by which you can play music for the public because you've paid a user fee.

- Our music mood changes over the course of the day. In the morning, we have an older crowd so we play easy listening. In the after-noon and evening, it's a younger, hipper crowd, and that's when we have on rock.

Helping Hands

The curse of the beauty professional is dry, cracked, and often bleeding hands from continued exposure to moisture and chemicals. The following ideas and suggestions may alert you to some products on the market that you didn't even know existed, but this is not, in any sense, an endorsement of these products, as we have not tested them ourselves. Have a look and ask your pharmacist and colleagues what they recommend.

◉ I like Aquaphor lotion. You can get it over the counter at most drugstores. It's popular among physicians for their own personal use. In fact, I have a client who's a dermatologist and she recommended it to me over any prescription stuff.

◉ Aquaphor's really good, but it's very heavy and greasy. Use cotton gloves at night or you'll wind up having to get new sheets. If you're looking for something good but not so greasy, try Eucerin. It's quality stuff.

◉ I find a lot of skin lotions and creams to be highly overpriced and don't see that much of a variation from one to the other. I make do with Vaseline at night, using cotton gloves, which makes a big difference.

◉ I've come across something that may be hard to find but it's worth the search. It's called Kerodex 71. It's nongreasy, invisible, and water-repellent, and you use it routinely for water work.

◉ I went through a whole lot of creams and salves and lotions before I found one that worked for me. It's called Ultra Mide 25. It used to be available only by prescription but now you can get it over the counter. I think a lot of the decision that goes into finding something to take care of these awful hands that so many of us have is trial and error. What works for some may not work for you. It's a matter of your body chemistry matching up with the chemistry of the product.

- I get by with Dermasil Dry Skin Treatment Lotion.

- If my hands are really suffering, I'll use A & D ointment. As you probably know, it's what takes care of diaper rash, so you'll probably find it in the baby section of the pharmacy. I rub it in, throw on some cotton gloves, and in the morning, my hands are smiling!

- I took over this girl's station after she left on a day's notice, and one of the things she left behind was this stuff called Gly-Miracle. Well, let me tell you, it was a miracle. I've never before or since had anything better. It's made by Palm Beach Products, and it's this amazing combination of aloe and vitamin E and glycerine and Irish moss and I don't know what else. But it works!

- I always keep a bottle of Sarana handy at work. It really helps with burning and itching.

- A bunch of us at our salon use a product called Sole Food. It's designed for feet, but our feeling is that feet usually take a lot more abuse than hands too, so if it would work on feet, it might work on hands, right? In fact, it works great. Not the best smell in the world, but I'd put limburger cheese all over my hands if that would help.

- ◎ Ever hear of Qtica's Intensive Hand Repair? Check it out. It's a professional skin care product designed for retail sales in the salon. It's magic on dry and cracked hands.

- ◎ I like a product called Rex-Eme. It has that overpowering eucalyptus-menthol smell, but it makes my hands feel so much better.

- ◎ Try cotton gloves at night and Bag Balm. Bag Balm is this expensive stuff that you can usually buy in certain hardware stores or at a farm supply store if you live in or near a rural area. It was designed to soothe the chapped udders of cows. Now can you imagine anything that gets more wear and tear than a cow's tender udder that's milked by a farmer's rough hands?

- ◎ To me, if it's got the word "natural" in it, I'm half-sold. I like Burt's Bees products. Everything Burt makes is delicious, but the hand cream has almond oil and beeswax in it. I could eat it with a spoon.

- ◎ If you're looking for top value, check out an item called Gardener's Hand Repair. I get it at

Trader Joe's. It's so good and there's no animal testing or anything like that.

◎ The Body Shop has my vote. Their Body Butter products are fantastic.

◎ My discovery is Aloe Vesta 2-in-1. It's great and it's cheap. You can get it at any of the big chain stores or they'll order it for you.

◎ I'm allergic to a lot of the chemicals we use, so I've turned to a protection called Acid Mantle. It's totally done the trick for me.

◎ On my doctor's advice, I take fish mineral oil in capsule form. I think it's helped quite a bit. I guess it helps attack the dry skin problem systemically.

Chapter 7

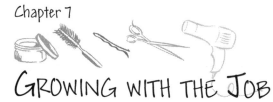

GROWING WITH THE JOB

I n the last few chapters, we have been hearing a lot of hands-on information about every-thing from the kind of shoes a cosmetologist should wear to the best lotion for chapped hands. But a big part of a cosmetologist's professional life has to do with meeting the more abstract demands of growing into the job. How do you stay fresh? How do you stay focused? Where do you look for creativity and inspiration? How do you integrate continuing education into your life?

In this chapter, we will also be talking about another area that requires a lot of growth for some people: retailing. Retailing is a major part of a cosmetologist's life and often, it is deeply feared.

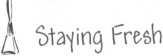

Staying Fresh

Sometime it feels like you're just stuck in a same old rut. Same old cuts, same old perms, same old clients asking for the same old thing, over and over again. This can drag you down, no doubt about it, but there are ways to counter that "same old" feeling.

◎ Be a "first-timer" every time you do something. It may be a trick of the mind but it's a good one. Every time you approach a task, act like it's your first time doing it. This may seem artificial at first, but it's a way of training your mind to stay alert, responsive, and engaged.

◎ I hear a lot of the young stylists in my shop going on about how "bored" they are. Everything has to feel like three minutes of excitement. Life isn't like that. If you get three minutes of excitement in a week, you're in good shape.

◎ I stay fresh by telling myself that every service I undertake is an opportunity for triumph or disaster. Now, realistically, 90 percent of what I do falls somewhere in between. But there's always the chance that I could soar or I could fail. I never know at the beginning what will happen at the end.

◎ Staying fresh has not been such a big issue for me, simply because I love what I'm doing. I

love the camaraderie of the salon, I love the relationships I make with clients, I love the
money, and most of all, I love the fact that I
make people happy. When people come in
looking one way and leave looking a whole lot
better, they get these smiles on their faces that
make my day, day after day after day.

◎ Okay, so may be you're going to think I'm a
terrible person because I'm not going to give
you a whole hearts-and-flowers spiel, but the
thing that keeps me fresh in this business is
knowing that I'm going to be making money.
Seriously, for me it's a "show me the money"
thing. I know that I am a highly skilled professional with highly marketable skills. I have advanced steadily and productively in this
business. I know that the more I work, the
more money I can make. When I'm tired and
feeling a little stale, I take some of that money
and I go off to Acapulco or I go scuba diving in
Belize or shopping in Paris and I feel recharged.
Shallow? Whatever!

◎ Look, you have to understand that this business is not just about proving yourself a genius
at styling. There aren't so many geniuses at
styling to be perfectly blunt about it. So, for
me, another way to stay fresh is to focus in on
the people I'm servicing. I like to really get to
know these people, and over the years, I've
formed very significant relationships with

them. We're not buddy-buddy, but we share interests; we talk about movies and plays and music and our kids and whether they've been to the new restaurant in town, and that kind of interaction does a lot to recharge me.

◎ If I feel like I'm getting into a ho-hum/hum-drum place, I play games. For instance, I time myself. Nobody knows I'm doing it but me. I say to myself, "Let's see just how fast you can get this one done." Now keep in mind that I'm not cutting any corners. It's very subtle. It's just fun for me to see if I can shave off a minute or two, purely for the challenge of it.

◎ I've never found the "freshness" issue to be an issue. Why? Because I've never had the same day two days in a row in this business. If you're really serious and in there, there are so many variables to keep your day fresh. There's interpersonal stuff in the salon, there's retailing, and there's education. Come on!

The Creativity Factor

Creativity, like health, is something that you need to work at to protect, preserve, and foster. The more you use your creativity, the more it grows. And what exactly is creativity? Some people define it as the ability to take existing objects and put them together in different ways so that they can serve a new purpose. Other people use a broader definition of creativity: the ability to generate new and useful ideas and solutions. Let's have a look at how your colleagues in the field view the issue of creativity.

◉ I find that creativity is spurred by an exchange of ideas. I like to brainstorm with other people. I do this in a couple of ways. I've always zeroed in on two or three people in the salon who I think are truly creative, and I recharge with them. We'll have coffee together or we might go to a museum or a concert after work some times, and talk about what we've seen and heard.

◉ One way I feel that I keep my creativity alive is by cultivating relationships with people outside the world of cosmetology. I number among my friends artists, writers, musicians, a biologist, a close friend who's an attorney, teachers, and from each of them I get a different view of the world. I think it's very important to get away from the "world as a salon" view of things.

◉ How do you stay creative? Surprise your mind every way you can think of. Take a different route to work. Walk or bike: the world will look entirely different to you. Eat dessert first. Or have breakfast for dinner at a diner. Pancakes in the evening will make your day feel different. And when your day feels different, it's one way to invite creativity in.

◎ I like to watch children. Fortunately, I have two of my own, but if I didn't, I'd borrow some for the day every now and then. Picasso said that every child is an artist and the problem for people is how to remain an artist after you've grown up. Kids are amazing because they haven't been told that they can't do things, so they look at a problem and they consider creative solutions all the time. Watch kids and think about how they play, and adapt some of their behavior to your own life. Get into the sensual pleasures of tactile experiences. As a child enjoys finger painting, let yourself go back to the pleasure you used to feel in running your hands through someone's hair.

◎ One way to hold onto your creativity is to make a time and a place for it. If you're running around every minute of the day, doing your job, picking up your dry-cleaning, running to the bank, or talking on the phone to your mother, you have to realize that you have not factored in your creativity time. Creativity does not emerge for most of us without a little help.

◎ Sometimes I imagine being in this Japanese teahouse in the middle of a bamboo grove and I think about how creative I would be if I could spend time in such a place. All these ideas and inspirations would just flow out of me. But I live in Danbury, Connecticut, and there are no bamboo groves to be had. But I have created a place in my house, small as it is, that I think of as my creativity space. I have a Japanese-style desk fountain that makes a lovely babbling noise, and a beautiful glossy jade plant. I sip green tea, and in those quiet and unrushed moments, I let my creative thoughts come to me. Sometimes they don't come, and I haven't lost anything. But those times when they do come, I've gained so much.

◎ Creativity is something you can really work at, and to a certain extent, learn. At least you can learn ways to cultivate it. There are many good books on the market about creativity and many places where you can attend workshops on the subject.

◎ I keep a daily journal. It's a place for me to focus my thoughts and to get in touch with the inner me. I write in it every night before I go to bed. Maybe just 10 minutes or so, but it's enough to stay in touch with the part of me that too easily can get tamped down by all the rigors and stresses of life.

◎ I think you can become a more creative person by being patient and letting creativity come to you, and especially by not judging yourself harshly. I took a drawing class because I wanted to be able to see people with new eyes. Our instructor, who was great, told us in the first class not to criticize ourselves. That's just a way of censoring your creativity, he said.

- You want to be more creative? Then create a more stimulating environment. Creativity often comes when you stimulate the senses by reading a poem, listening to music, or inhaling the scent of a rose geranium. Any of these activities, and, of course, hundreds more, can be a sensual spur to igniting your creative spark.

- Why do some people have a problem with creativity? Because they allow obstacles to be placed in their path such as an irrational fear of criticism, a lack of confidence, or an overemphasis on the negative stresses in your life. Those obstacles need to be cleared away. Lock them up in a safe box and don't let them out!

- Relaxation is a good lubricant to get the creative juices going. Quiet relaxation for the most part, like meditation, or handwork such as knitting or quilting, or quiet exercise like a long walk or swimming. These are all ways of helping yourself make room for creativity.

- Learn to recognize your "creative time." We all walk around with a certain internal biological clock. Some of us are night people; some of us are morning people. If you're a morning person, don't sit down to write a poem at midnight when you're ready to fall off your feet. Go with the flow of who you really are.

- Bust out of the box. Smash your routines. If you're used to doing things one way, do them another way. Routines used indiscriminately can lead to a bureaucratic frame of mind, which is totally antithetical to creativity.

◎ Develop an interest in a wide variety of things and start enjoying the experience of learning about things in depth. I feel like I've remained intellectually alive and creative by always making myself learn about things. I became very interested in Russian Easter Egg art and I found out everything I could about it. Same for harpsichord music. Same for making beer (that was another obsession of mine for a while). I really enjoy the stimulation of becoming an "expert" at different things.

◎ I stay creative by making big changes in my life. I've organized my life around this principle. I've stayed single, and being in the cosmetology field, I can move anywhere and everywhere I want. And that's exactly what I've done. Two years in Brazil, a year in Vancouver, a year in London, two years in Capetown. I know that's not a lifestyle that would work for everyone, but do I have a creativity problem? Hardly. Boredom is not in my vocabulary.

◎ When you come down to it, creativity and education go hand in hand. If you feel like you're getting stale and old hat, find a new way to do something. There's so much out there in terms of educational opportunities that there's no excuse not to do just that.

 ## Continuing Education

Most cosmetologists we spoke to emphasized the critical need for those in the field to remain committed to the practice of continuing education.

◉ Because the field is continually changing, you need to pursue education for now and for always. I tell young stylists to figure on no less than 40 hours a year of continuing education. But, of course, the more the better.

◉ Education is key in this business. If you don't keep moving, you fall behind. It's as simple as that. Clients are becoming more and more sophisticated. They read magazines; they watch television. They know what they want, and if they ask you for something and you don't know how to give it to them, they're going to go find it from somebody else.

◉ For some people, money is the bottom line, and they'll ask me, "Well, how much should we *have* to spend on continuing education?" I reply, "You don't *have* to spend anything; that's your choice. But, if I were you, I'd factor in about $1,000 a year on continuing education."

Now do you think that's such an exorbitant sum of money to invest in yourself and to acquire skills that allow you to move higher and higher up the ladder?

◎ A young stylist doesn't have to spend a fortune to brush up his skills with continuing education. Manufacturers are always offering free classes, and a young stylist can earn points in the salon by researching some of these educational opportunities and bringing them to the attention of the salon manager. That's called initiative!

◎ I had a young stylist in the salon I own who spent his own money to go to a hair show. He came back with some great techniques that he offered to teach, for free, to his coworkers. I rewarded him (and made up his out-of-pocket expenses) by paying him for his teaching.

◎ Belonging to trade associations is another good way for a stylist to get into an education frame of mind. With such a membership, you'll get trade journals and newsletters that will clue you in to what's happening out there, and that will let you know where you can go for important educational opportunities. Your membership will also avail you of all the new and important information around regulations, insurance, and other important things you need to know.

- The big upscale salons in the cities and suburbs often will pay the way for stylists who want to partake of educational opportunities, or at the very least, they'll be visited on a regular basis by product educators from manufacturers who offer all kinds of free seminars and workshops. But what do you do if you're working in a rural setting? Say you're in a small town in a county that has maybe a dozen shops altogether. Well, one thing you can do in that situation is network. The shops can band together and pool money for the necessary educational opportunities. Maybe you can all go in together on some important educational videos and you can make a time for people to come together collectively to watch them. That kind of interconnection can be so positive.

- Friendly competition is a stimulus to continuing education. If I'm in a town with just a few salons and I see that my competitor across the street is doing better than I am, I want to find out what he's doing and I want to learn how to do it. That kind of competition is not a destructive thing; on the contrary, it can be a really valuable wake-up call. Just the thing you need to get you up and going!

- A lot of people are finding technical education available on the Internet to be very useful. You can log onto any number of sites and get graphic, 3-D representations of how to do various techniques. It's not for everyone because some people need that in-the-flesh, hands-on thing, but for other people, it's a free way to learn and a way that can be incorporated into almost anyone's schedule.

◉ I don't find the Internet useful in terms of learning techniques but I do check regularly with a bunch of different sites where I can chat and engage in idea exchanges.

◉ Don't think upscale salons are the only ones who get behind continuing education. The value chains also regularly provide in-house modules on a variety of topics like self-esteem and communication skills, as well as regular visits from product educators.

◉ When you're being considered for a job, you can explore whether continuing education can be factored into your overall benefits package. It's a nice perk that might make the difference if you're trying to decide between a couple of different offers.

◉ Hair shows are an exciting way to learn some new and glitzy stuff, with the emphasis often on the glitzy. The learning opportunities on the main trade show floor are often too geared to what's showy and won't translate very effectively to what you really need when you get back home. Better you should check out some of the small, behind-closed-doors seminars that are usually orbiting around the main event.

- I used to bring some of the young stylists with me to hair shows, but I found that a lot of them acted like kids on a field trip. Maybe they'd take in a class or two, but the rest of the time they were too busy running around looking for freebies. Now I've come to the decision that the responsibility for continuing education should be on the stylists' shoulders. Yes, it's an expense but it's also a way for the stylist to invest in herself for the coming years. And nothing breeds commitment like shelling out your own money.

The Joy of Retailing

For many cosmetologists, the act of retailing is something they have to grow into. It can also be an avenue of continued personality development and job satisfaction. Nothing is more exciting than discovering that you have a real aptitude for something you never even thought you'd be good at!

- Some people see retailing as the gravy. There are times when I see it as the meat. It really makes the difference between a job and a career by which you can be well remunerated.

- A lot of cosmetologists feel that they "just can't sell." For some reason, they seem to think that selling a jar of conditioner is going to turn them into a used-car salesman. What they don't realize is that there's a good and right and honorable way to sell anything, including used cars, and that you are actually doing your salon and your clients a favor by selling them quality products.

◎ Some people are really hung up about selling and it's important to overcome this hang-up. You don't have to be pushy or aggressive or obnoxious to be successful salesperson. While certainly there are salespeople like that, there are also very helpful and knowledgeable sales professionals who care about their customers above all else.

◎ There are certain basic principles behind the act of selling. The most important is that you are selling yourself. Nobody is going to buy a candy bar from somebody they don't like or trust. So how do you begin to sell yourself? Your start by feeling good about who you are and what you're selling.

◎ It's crucial to be totally familiar with the items you're trying to sell. You need to know all of the strengths and any drawbacks, if they exist. If the strengths are really strong and if the drawbacks are comparatively minor, then alert the buyer to those drawbacks. Have everything up front and out in the open. That's a way to promote trust between the seller and the buyer.

◎ Knowing your product is absolutely essential. That means doing your homework. Virtually all of the distributors offer product classes for the salon. These range from basic fundamentals to really sophisticated advanced techniques. Tell the educators what you hope to achieve from their classes. You want them to give you merchandising ammunition—why should someone buy this product?—and to suggest ways to close the sale. They'll know what you're talking about.

◉ Trust is very important in the buyer-seller contract. Would you want to be sold something that wasn't very good or that you didn't really need? Obviously not. Well then, don't try to do that to someone else. You can thrive in the retailing area simply by selling the things you believe in to the people who need them.

◉ You want to customize your selling approach to each and every one of your clients. Customize and personalize. I'm not just talking about a hard sell versus a soft sell approach, although that's part of it. Some of your clients need to be pushed and they won't resent it; others will chafe at a hard sell. You have to know that about them. But you should also customize your approach by knowing the specifics in your clients' lives. "Mrs. Jones, you're going to Florida next month. You ought to think about picking up some of this new conditioner that works wonders on hair that's been exposed to the sun and other elements."

That's the kind of customizing I'm talking about.

- Selling is a dance and selling is a dialogue. You want to ask questions that will help you determine a client's needs, and then you want to lead, firmly, like any good dancer does.

- Pictures tell a thousand words. Whenever possible, demonstrate your product.

- The most important part of the retailing process is what salespeople call "closing the sale." It's that precise psychological moment when the buyer is ready to buy. When that happens, stop selling. In other words, don't oversell. Simply reassure the buyer that he has made the right decision.

- In terms of selling, nothing is more magical than a promotion or a discount or a sale. The more you get into retailing, the more you'll realize that. "We have a special this month on . . ." are golden words with which to start a retailing conversation.

- Put the product in the client's hands. Let her touch it/smell it/taste it if she wants. At the very least, put the product in the client's view range. Sometimes I'll go into shops and they'll have the products way above viewing level. Why are products placed above clients' heads?

And why are they behind glass in some places like a "No Touch" museum?

◎ If the retail area in your salon is sloppy or poorly thought out, your selling job is going to be ten times as hard. Approach the powers that be about improving the lighting if necessary, and, of course, everything should be kept scrupulously clean. The selling area should also have plenty of product; it shouldn't look like it's a going-out-of-business sale. There's an old adage in the retailing business: Show more, sell more.

◎ Don't forget signs. Your salon selling area should be clearly and plentifully signed. HAIR CARE . . . SKIN CARE . . . NAIL CARE. The client should be able to walk into the selling area and focus in on the products. Prices, too, should be visible on everything. Some clients will never ask what something costs, and that means that if they don't know the price, you may automatically lose the sale.

◎ Remember that in most cases, you are selling professional products that cannot be bought in a supermarket or drug store. Be informed as to the ways in which these professional products are superior to the other brands.

◎ As a stylist, you're going to be involved in another significant arena of sales: ticket upgrading, also known as upselling. This refers to the selling of salon services. You want to become skilled at that because it means a lot in terms of increased revenues for you and the salon. As is the case when you are selling retail products, selling salon services depends a lot on your awareness of who the client is and what is happening in her life. "Mrs. Jones, you've got a wedding coming up, right? Did you ever think about having a professional makeup consultation?" Selling is all about persuasion, and persuasion works best when you have a clear sense of who you're dealing with.

◉ When it comes to ticket upgrading, I tell my stylists to keep three guidelines in mind:

1. offer at least one additional service idea per client

2. alert all of your clients to any special promotions or sales that the salon is running

3. describe to the client in juicy detail exactly how the service you're recommending is going to benefit them (for instance, their hair will be shinier, easier to style, less tangled, easier to maintain, or whatever).

◉ As a manager, I feel that it is very important for all salons to have ongoing training in retailing. This kind of training should focus on effective consultations, the art of closing, and cooperation between the front desk, the client, and the stylist. There are lots of great videos out there on selling that should be brought in for the salon staff. The message should be that everyone in the salon needs to get behind selling together!

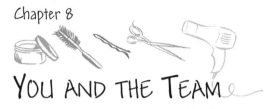

Chapter 8

YOU AND THE TEAM

o you remember being graded in elementary school on a category called "Works and Plays Well with Others?" You could get an Excellent, a Good, a Satisfactory, or an Unsatisfactory. Well, guess what? We're *still* being graded on our skills in that area. Every day of our lives, people are looking at us—our bosses, our managers, our coworkers, our clients—and they are judging whether we are excellent, good, okay, or really not so good at getting along with other people.

Some people are blessed with sunny personalities and the ability to attract others into their orbit. These people are natural leaders who manage to convince others to do things their way; they are sought out and sought after, whether the context is professional or social. Other people are quiet, reserved, or even shy. Entering a group is always something they have to "rehearse." Their interactions are rarely spontaneous, but can still be successful and satisfying. Still others have significant problems fitting into a group altogether.

Personalities are a complicated issue, but fortunately we can all learn new and useful ways to interact with others. In this chapter, we will be hearing from your fellow cosmetologists on how they have improved their interrelationships, with specific attention paid to such matters as conflict resolution, dealing with difficult people, mentoring, and more.

 ## Communication Basics

Relationships start with communication. If you can't make your wants and needs known, or if you can't hear the wants and needs of others, you're going to have a hard time being part of a team.

◉ The first thing people have to realize is that *everything* is communication, not just the words that come out of your mouth: the expression on your face, the way you make eye contact, your body language. All that stuff telegraphs messages just as fast, if not faster, than words.

So if you want someone to get a message—or maybe even more important, if you *don't* want them to get a message—keep your body language in mind.

◉ When you're talking about communication, it's important to keep in mind cultural differences. In some cultures, looking down, for instance, is a sign of deference or respect. On a job interview, however, if you look down, people may think you've got something to hide.

◉ My pet peeve has to do with people who don't observe space barriers. Good communication cannot occur when somebody is invading your personal space. I read somewhere once that family, lovers, and close friends are comfortable standing about a foot apart. Everyone else should observe the 4-foot to 12-foot minimum.

◉ Good communication has a lot to do with the quality of your voice. If you're strident or if you mumble, that gives people a message about who you are. Maybe the wrong message. Have a friend give you a "voice test." Find out if your voice needs to be softened or strengthened, and work on it. I remember reading in high school about some Greek philosopher who learned to speak with marbles in his mouth. We ought to be able to improve the way we speak without having to go to such lengths.

◉ It helps me to recognize that some people have attention problems. I'm a manager and I've had stylists working for me who were great one-on-one. But put them in a busy room and they wouldn't hear a word I was saying. They're so busy scanning to see what's going on around them that it's like talking to a wall. You've got to alert them to this problem—it's called "selective attention"—and help them with it.

◉ As a manager, I find it useful to consider the various communication styles I see among my staff. Some people have what I call a "Selling Style:" they like to touch and feel and talk. Others are the ones I call "The Thinkers" who tend to be guarded but may also be great problem-solvers. Then you've got the "Relaters" who interact warmly and who really seem to care about other people. I try to identify each person who works for me along these lines and use them where they are most effective.

◉ Not everybody realizes that they can become better listeners. There are listening skills to learn and listening issues to become aware of. For instance, maybe the person you're talking to has a hearing deficit. We had a stylist who didn't seem to listen very well at all. We urged him to get a hearing test and it turned out that he had significant hearing loss from the years he'd spent in a rock band! All the while, people in the salon thought he was just someone who never paid any attention when, in fact, he had a real physiological problem.

- A big part of communication is asking good questions. Some people never seem to ask questions. Others are full of them. I like the latter. Asking questions shows curiosity and interest, and a quality of being present in the moment. In fact, not only do I encourage my staff to ask questions, but I teach them how to get into a questioning mode. I advise them to look at any given situation with question words in mind like who, what, where, when, why, and how.

- I try to correct the mispronunciations of people who work for me. I know not everyone appreciates it, but I can't resist. Why should somebody go through life saying "drownded" instead of "drowned" or "akst" instead of "asked?" What I do is lie: I say, "I used to make that mistake, too." I bring up the issue gently and out of real feeling for the other person.

Personality and Attitude

Let's face it. If you are a cosmetologist, you are dealing day to day with people. If you don't like to deal with people, another field might make more sense. In assessing how you are with people, it's helpful to make a distinction between personality and attitude. One can have an introverted personality (shy, quiet, reserved) and yet have a positive attitude about other people. Conversely, one can be extroverted (outgoing, center-of-attention type) and yet have a negative attitude about others. Attitude, on the other hand, is influenced or even formed by our environment: all the things we learn and take away from parents, teachers, peers, even books and movies. We many not be able to change a characteristic that we were born with but we can change our attitude.

◎ Coming from a long line of passive women, I had to learn to be assertive. My mentor helped me understand how I could stand up for myself and ask what I wanted without sounding like I was complaining or being aggressive.

◎ A guy I worked with early on in my career taught me the secret of assertiveness. It's a three-step process, he explained. The key phrases are "I feel," "I want," "I will." For instance, *I feel* I'm being taken advantage of in this situation. *I want* to be valued as a person. *I will* make it known that I do not allow myself to be treated disrespectfully.

◎ There's a four-letter word that I like to introduce to all of the young people who come to work in our salon: *tact*. It's enlightening to some to learn that you don't have to say everything that comes into your head, and that you can be straightforward and honest without being harsh and critical.

◎ Reframing is an important concept to help you adjust your attitude. Reframing essentially allows you to change the meaning of an event. For instance, you might perceive a criticism from your boss as a put-down or even a devastating ego blow. Reframing lets you put the brakes on those feelings. When you slow down, you can see the experience as an opportunity to learn.

◎ Don't make an opera out of every little thing. To resist that impulse is something that comes with maturity, but it's never too early to start learning. Let a coworker's inappropriate comment roll off your back. Before you know it, you'll forget it even happened.

◎ I look for sensitivity in a person, someone who knows when to speak and knows when to listen. Being a sensitive person doesn't mean being a doormat. Sensitivity is a strength, not a weakness.

◎ Practice listening. If your boss calls you in to discuss some shortcoming he sees in your performance, don't rush to your defense. Try saying absolutely nothing for a good long while and really listen.

- When you get good at "basic listening," you can advance to "reflective listening." This has worked like a charm for me in terms of getting people to see me as a positive member of the salon community. Basically, I listen to what people have to say and then I give it back to them. For instance, if they say, "I don't know if you are up to this . . . ," I'll say something like, "It seems you're unsure of my capabilities." People like to hear what they have said returned to them, and it almost always winds up building toward a real dialogue.

- If you read anything about business skills and how to handle yourself in a professional situation, you'll probably come across the concept of "mirroring." Imagine, for instance, that you have a very nervous, first-time client who's come in for a coloring. In the course of the consultation, you "mirror" back to her things about herself: the way she answers a question with a question, let's say, holds her head, or crosses her legs. This is a very fast and effective way of building trust.

- In order to present the kind of positive attitude that will make you a valuable part of a team, you've got to learn how to receive criticism. As a manager, I see people receiving criticism in a variety of ways. Some withdraw; some rationalize. Some project, trying to blame others. All of these responses are normal defense mechanisms, but you have to get beyond them and find more positive ways to handle negative feedback.

◉ When I get negative feedback, I have to first consider from whom it's coming. Do I respect this person? If not, I pay only so much attention. If I do respect this person, then I listen and ask for specific information. Some people offer criticism in only general terms, and that doesn't help me very much.

◉ I have this to say about criticism: let it sink in. Don't feel you have to respond to it right away, or at all. Take your time and mull it over.

◉ I always go for the "second opinion." For instance, if a boss says to me, "You're disorganized," I'll canvass my family and friends. "Am I disorganized? Have you noticed this about me? Just how disorganized would you say I am?" It's a reality test, and even if it hurts, it's important to know the truth.

◉ Giving negative feedback can be as hard as getting it. An important rule to remember is to criticize people only on those matters you think they can change. If someone is clearly not a genius, it does no good to say, "You're not very smart." But things like organization and neatness, and a sense of responsibility, are qualities that almost all of us can improve on to some degree or other.

◎ When giving criticism, make sure to package it as positively and constructively as possible, and always criticize specific behaviors, not personality. In other words, instead of saying, "You're so sloppy," say something like, "I would appreciate it if you could be more careful when placing the soiled towels in the container."

◎ The message that I try to establish in the salon I manage is that everyone should be treated with respect. And you don't have to like someone to treat that person with respect. You just have to realize that you are part of a team and that person is bringing revenue into the salon.

◎ Practice being neutral like Switzerland. Chances are, down the road, someone is going to try to pull you into a conflict and get you to "pick a side." Resist it. And resist the impulse to gossip with others about people. Like spitting out a car window, it will only come back to hit you in the face.

◎ Don't take everything so personally. Sometimes, people have a bad day and you just happen to be there at the wrong time. Don't assume that a brusque word or a look was really intended as an assassination attempt on your life. If you're feeling weird about how someone's acted toward you, get that person alone in a quiet corner and ask her about it. You may quickly find out, to your relief, that it's a whole lot of nothing.

◎ Always, always, always *keep your private life private*! Some people confuse camaraderie in the workplace with real intimacy. Don't fall into that trap. Save intimacy for your intimate friends and family members you trust. Loose lips sink ships and can make your life miserable if you've told somebody something about yourself or about someone else (particularly another coworker or a client) that you shouldn't have.

◎ Be concerned, not only with your own success but also with the success of others. Stay a little later or come in a little earlier to help out a teammate.

◎ Pitch in whenever you can. Don't worry about your "place" or your "standing." Sometimes, it makes sense for everyone to help with appointments or even to fold towels. Remember, you're part of a team. All for one and one for all!

◎ Be generous with your knowledge. I once had an aunt who made the world's greatest lasagna. She would never share the recipe with anyone. When she died, the lasagna went to the grave with her. Don't be like my aunt. If you know something, share it. This will make you a valued and important member of the team.

 ## Conflict Resolution

Regardless of where you work, you are bound to come into conflict somewhere along the way with a manager, a coworker, a client, or any and all of the above. The way you handle and resolve conflict will have a lot to do with your ultimate success in a job and in life in general.

◎ Sure, there are techniques to help you deal with conflict but there are no real shortcuts. The foundation for healthy conflict resolution begins with you. When you fully understand who you are and what makes you tick, then you can begin to understand others.

◎ Keep in mind that healthy and positive conflict resolution is not going to be taking place in an atmosphere of mistrust and insecurity. If you're working in a shop with a lot of "top-down" nuttiness, then you have to expect conflict to rear its ugly head on every level.

◎ To resolve conflict successfully, you have to have an understanding of how anger works and how various individuals deal with it. Some people grow up in homes where it is taboo to be angry, and they internalize their anger or become so passive that their aggression comes out in lots of little ways. Other people are of a road rage variety and may be completely inappropriate in the way they give vent to their anger. You need to know the anger styles of your coworkers and proceed accordingly when you have a conflict with any one of them.

◉ A lot of conflict is best resolved by the classic tactic of turning the other cheek. Usually, people who give you a lot of grief turn out to be very insecure, unhappy people. You don't have to get down to their level. Be the big one, even if officially, you are below them on the pecking order.

◉ I think the most effective tool I use when I'm in a conflict is to address the other party with his name. When I say, "What is the problem, John?" or "What can we do to work this out, Mary?" it shows that I see these individuals as people and it defuses their anger toward me.

◉ My grandfather used to say something that I carry with me to this day: "It is easy to make an enemy; it is harder to keep a friend." I like that saying because it conveys how quickly a relationship can sour, how precious a good relationship is, and how difficult it can be to remedy it when it's been damaged.

◉ When two wolves get into a fight, one makes itself submissive and shows its jugular to its adversary. This display usually puts an end to the aggression. I've found it useful to adapt that wolf behavior to conflicts that come my way. I will say to the other person, "You know, I really feel I could use your help to figure a way out of this mess." When I do this, the other person rushes to help me and I never feel I am taken advantage of.

◎ I laugh. Not necessarily with the person I'm having the problem with, but I find somewhere in my day and life to have a good guffaw. If I'm having a conflict with someone, I'll go out to lunch with my friend Sandy who I know is an absolute riot. She does these amazing imperson-ations of people we work with. After an hour with Sandy, I'm feeling no pain. It's like nitrous oxide, and when I go back to work and see the person who's been giving me a hard time, it just doesn't seem to matter so much anymore.

◎ Listen, listen, listen. Then listen some more. Some people, in a conflict, are so anxious to state their case that they don't even hear what the other person has to say. And if you come up against such a person, you can gently sug-gest that they listen to you.

◎ The best kind of conflict resolution? To me, it's building relationships so that when conflict comes along, you're ready for it. I build rela-tionships by being honest, by giving people positive and constructive feedback, and by caring about them.

◎ Never say or do anything in haste and never, ever, write anything down! I think one of the worst inventions known to mankind is e-mail, in the sense that too many people, when they're angry, will go to their computer and jot off a furious note. Well, that e-mail becomes a historical record of your anger that you would rather not see again when you're feeling better. Use self-control in all your dealings and don't shoot off (or write off) at the mouth!

◎ Before, after, and, if possible, during a conflict, share a good feeling with the other person. Tell them something good about themselves. By doing so, you acknowledge the conflict but place it in the larger context of a fuller relationship.

◎ Go for a walk. Breathe deeply. Eat a doughnut. Do something to break the chain of the anger. Then you can go back and look at the situation differently, and decide what to do next.

◎ I think the key to conflict resolution is a commitment to resolving the conflict. You and the other person have to be on the same page. Make it a page that says, "We *will* get beyond this. We *must* get beyond this."

◎ In order to resolve the conflict, it's important to ask yourself what you're looking for. For some people, it's an apology. The apology is like this pot of gold at the end of the rainbow. I tell people not to be so focused on apologies. Focus on coexistence instead.

◎ When you're trying to iron out a conflict with someone, always stay in the present. Always. Never bring up a whole history of slights and insensitivities. Once you start doing that, things will spiral out of control.

You and Your Manager

Your relationship with your manager is an important and complex one. Here are some guidelines that your colleagues thought you might find useful.

◎ Don't always go to the manager looking to have your problems solved. She is just another highly fallible member of the human race. When you need to speak with your manager about a problem you're having, try your best to think about some possible solutions beforehand. It'll make a great impression.

◎ Your manager is there to help. Don't pretend you know how to do something or how to solve some problem if you don't really. Be open and honest about the gaps in your knowledge base and your manager will help you fill them in.

- Nobody likes a tattletale. It was true in kindergarten and it's true now in the real world. If you're having a legitimate problem with a coworker and don't feel that you can successfully resolve it yourself, then you can seek out your manager for input and mediation. But you have to approach the manager with a real desire to solve the problem, not just for the opportunity to vent.

- Expect to hear constructive criticism from your manager and receive it as well as you can. It's her job to give it; it's your job to receive it.

- Your employee evaluation or job review is a very important experience in your work life. Ask your manager for a copy of the evaluation form that he will be using and look it over carefully to make sure you understand it. You might want to check out the form some weeks or even months in advance of your review so that you can chart yourself and have a good sense of how you're doing when the review rolls around.

- As a manager, I tell my stylists to evaluate themselves. Check out the form and then rate yourself as objectively as you can. If you do this in advance of the review, there's a good chance that you and your manager may be on the same page in your regard. Or, at least, you'll have a relatively intelligent basis from which to argue in your behalf.

◉ I advise my stylists to write down any thoughts or questions they might have before the review. I tell them not to be shy. If you want to talk money, fine. If you want to be considered for a promotion, fine. Just lay it all out for me. This requires some planning on their parts.

. . . And Now You Have an Assistant

Having an assistant can be an adjustment. Here are some thoughts on how to make the most of that relationship:

- Start with small stuff.

- Have the assistant hand you tools or fill out information on cards.

- Let the assistant follow you around.

- Introduce the assistant to the customers.

- Maybe the assistant can work up toward shampoos or blow-drying that you finish off.

- Be an educator and mentor to your assistant.

Dealing with Difficult People

It is possible to find yourself embroiled in a conflict with almost anyone, but usually these conflicts can be resolved easily enough. Chances are, however, that you have encountered downright difficult people, whether they be coworkers, management, or clients, and you may be wondering how best to deal with them.

◉ I compliment these people. Relentlessly. I have this one client we'll call Mrs. Jones. Mrs. Jones is the world's worst pain but I flatter her every inch of the way. "Mrs. Jones, don't you look lovely today." "Mrs. Jones, yellow is your color." "Oh, Mrs. Jones, you've got such a fascinating life." This may sound phony, but it's no skin off my back and it keeps everyone happy.

◉ One of my pals in the salon had a huge blowout with another stylist, a woman I'll call Brenda. Now Brenda is a troublemaker, a real spoiler kind of personality. My friend was fuming. I said, "Hold it right there. Send Brenda flowers instead." "What?!" my friend cried. "You heard me." After we went back and forth a little, my friend did as I suggested and it worked like magic. At first, my friend thought that to send flowers would be an admission of guilt, but I told her that the more important thing was for her to look like a peacemaker in everyone else's eyes. That is exactly what happened.

◎ When it comes to dealing with difficult people, simply staying out of their line of view is the best strategy. It might sound really simplistic, but if you regard avoidance as a real technique, you'll see how effective it is. I know in my salon that we have one person who's a real witch, and you'd be surprised how many people, on their own steam, fly right into her orbit.

◎ I think a little sympathy and patience goes a long way toward dealing with difficult people. Some of my friends call me "The Saint" because they know I have this attitude, but I'm comfortable with it. I feel that difficult people often have difficult lives or have had difficult childhoods, and I try to forgive them as much as I can.

Little Things Mean a Lot

There is much to be said for the kind gesture, the show of concern, and the external motivation.

◎ I'm very concerned with team-building. We do things in our shop like celebrate birthdays. Whenever it's somebody's special day, as soon as that person comes into the shop, we play Destiny's Child's "Birthday" full blast, we put this funky tiara on the person's head, and it's a hoot. Everyone loves it. And we have cake and candles, too. You'd be amazed how far something like that goes toward team-building.

◎ I wouldn't dream of a salon without a suggestion box. Some of my staff, when they first got here, were skeptical, like it was silly to have a suggestion box. But you should see how they get into it. And some of our best ideas have come out of that little box.

◎ I always like to look for ways to empower people. Take music, for instance. I've worked in salons where the music really becomes a control issue, and if you don't play your cards right, you might wind up listening to music you don't like all day long. In our salon, we've got a satellite dish. It's wonderful. You get 100 channels that play everything from rock to pop to jazz to country to rap to disco to opera and more. There's nothing to store and nothing to pilfer. Every day, we let someone else pick the music. That means one day you have to listen to a lot of stuff you might not like, but you know your day is coming.

◎ Christmas is a big time around here. Not only do people get their bonuses, but everyone— and I mean absolutely everyone—gets a nice present (and I mean a *nice* present). I've heard of salons where people do a Christmas grab bag, too, and that sounds nice. Maybe we'll try it here.

◉ Incentives are a big part of what makes a happy team. That's just the way it is. And salons have to give real, careful, creative thought to how they are going to provide those incentives. In our salon, for instance, we've instituted a no-tipping policy. We collectively agreed that tipping was not a gesture that fit with the kind of professional image we were looking to project. Now we're making up for no more tips with other kinds of incentives like really good prizes for the best retailing performance and things like that.

◉ One incentive we use in our salon is flex-time. It lets you work a five-day week in four days. Everyone loves it. We've even been turning away good stylists who are looking for that kind of perk. That extra day is like the little vacation that comes every week. The pause that refreshes!

◉ Salons can piggyback on distributors for perks. There are always little things like T-shirts and totes to be given away, or, thinking more substantially, things like free passes to hair shows.

◉ I own a salon and I get a lot of great perks for my staff by bartering with customers. We cut the hair of people who own restaurants, jewelry stores, and clothing stores, and in exchange for free hair services, I get a steady stream of really good gift certificates to their establishments that I use as a continuous stream of freebies, rewarding everything from "most sales of the week" to "best attendance or punctuality" to "lucky number" type things.

The Mentor System

When we were little, our heroes were firemen or nurses or whoever. Now, as adults, our heroes are people we can look up to and who embody those qualities, professional and personal, that we wish to emulate. These people are called mentors, and being lucky enough to have one—or to be one—can make a world of difference.

◉ The mentoring relationship is so valuable for both parties. It's a way for the mentor to give back. In the past, you might have been mentored. Now it's your turn.

◉ The mentor relationship is really a two-way street. It's not just about the mentor teaching the mentee. I've learned a lot from my mentees.

◉ This may sound self-serving, and I don't mean it to, but mentoring someone is often a way for the mentor to look good in the eyes of management. Being able to help groom talent is an important skill to bring to the team, and it won't go unrecognized.

◎ I find mentoring a way to review and refresh my own knowledge base. Each time I teach, even in the relatively informal setting of a mentoring relationship, I go back to the material and that way, I hold on to it.

◎ Mentoring is energizing. A lot of what we have to fight against in this business is the "same old, same old." Mrs. Smith comes in asking for the same old flip she's been wearing forever. With mentoring, you're down in the trenches with new, fresh, unjaded blood. That helps keep me fresh, too.

◎ If you're being mentored, then *listen*. Don't talk: listen. That doesn't mean you shouldn't ask questions—in fact, you should—but it's not the sound of your own voice that you're looking to hear on this particular go-round.

◎ Neither mentors or mentees should expect to come away from the relationship with a fast friendship. If it happens, it happens, but that's not the reason for the relationship. The relationship is there for a purpose—a learning purpose—and that's what you need to understand.

◎ Like anyone in a teaching capacity, mentors should teach to a large extent by using positive reinforcement. Harsh criticism has no place in the mentoring relationship and can quickly end one.

◉ As a salon owner, I know how hard it is to find talented and reliable stylists. I never mentored until recently, but now I feel that by going back to my beauty school and mentoring a student, it's a good way to source stylists for the future.

◉ The dropout rate in this industry is outrageous. Students get out of beauty school in something like six months and then they're on their own. A mentor can be the safety net to keep that young stylist from bailing out of cosmetology.

When it comes to building a positive atmosphere within a salon, an important element is the kind of benefits being offered. Stylists and management alike should look at the following "wish list" and check it against the standards they have been living with:

◉ Health insurance

◉ Sick pay

◉ Paid vacation

◉ Retirement plans

◉ Security of employment

- Personal days

- Continuing education opportunities

- Promoting from within into jobs beyond the chair (that is, management, education, marketing, and the like)

- Flexible schedule

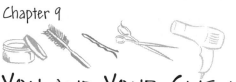

Chapter 9

YOU AND YOUR CLIENTS

You can be the very best stylist in the world, but that is not going to count for a lot unless you have clients. And the secret to getting and keeping clients goes beyond simply being a talented stylist. The stylists who manage to get and keep clients are usually good communicators.

Think about it. In a large or even average-sized city, a prospective client will have a lot of options when it comes to choosing a stylist. True, the client will look for a stylist with talent, but let's face it: there are plenty of talented stylists around. That means that other criteria will enter into a client's choice of which stylist to go with. The flexibility of the stylist, the stylist's capacity to hear the client's wishes, the ambiance that the stylist creates all work together to make a positive or negative experience for the client. In this chapter, we will be hearing from stylists about what works and what doesn't when it comes to getting and keeping clients.

The Relationship

Like any relationship, the one between stylist and client should be based on a strong foundation of respect and strong ethical values.

◉ I know a lot of stylists who act like their clients are their best friends. It always raises my antennae. I can have really warm feelings toward my clients and value them as human beings, but I decided early on to draw my friends from a whole other pool. I feel like it's a conflict of interest to turn a client into a friend. Then they'll start telling you personal things and it will break down the professionalism that must always be central to the relationship.

◉ Some people see the stylist-client relationship as being cut from the same cloth as the bartender-customer relationship. In other words, the stylist is there to hear your problems. I do everything I can to discourage that. To me, it's a false intimacy that only backfires in the long run.

◎ I'm a basically sympathetic and empathetic person, as I think most stylists should be, because, as stylists, we deal with a lot of personal material. A person's self-image, which is what we're dealing with, is deeply personal, after all. But talking about someone's eyes or nose or mouth or hair is different than talking about someone's husband or mother or daughter.

◎ We've all had this kind of experience: Mrs. Jones sits down in the chair and starts to pour out her tale of woe. Her husband's cheating on her; her daughter was picked up on a DWI; she's got a mole she doesn't like the looks of. Here's what I do. Before I've got everyone in the salon listening and taking notes, I get Mrs. Jones a beverage and I take her to a private part of the salon. I tell her that I'm sorry she's having troubles right now, but I think she really should view the salon visit as a time when she can get away from all that, and just relax and receive services that feel good. That's what I'm here for. And you know what? Usually the client is happy to follow my advice.

◎ Confidentiality is the bedrock of the stylist-client relationship. Going around telling other people what your client tells you is like tales told out of school. You will lose clients in a snap and you won't replace them in a snap either, once word gets around that you have breached someone's confidence.

◉ The dialogue that I enjoy with my clients is not
personal, but that doesn't mean it isn't warm,
engaged, and fun. We can talk about good
books we've read, good films we've seen, great
recipes, wonderful little hotels in Paris, and so
forth and so on. That's a lot different than air-
ing the family's dirty laundry. Friendly but not
personal. That's the key.

Client Communication

The communication basics we discussed in
Chapter 8 apply here as well. As with all commu-
nications, those you have with your clients
should take into account such factors as body language, cultural differences, appropriate space and
distance, tone of voice, and so on. But the communication you have with a client is even more
complex than the communication you have with
your coworkers, managers, and employers, and
stylists need to be aware of the special circumstances that affect this communication.

Meeting and Greeting

First impressions count for a lot. When meeting a
new client, you only will have a certain window
of opportunity during which to make a favorable
impression. And the work of making a favorable
impression doesn't end after that first visit. Treat
every visit as a first visit and remember that
clients are coming to you for services for which

they are paying their hard-earned cash. Treat them accordingly.

◎ Smile, please. Even if you're not having such a great day, you still have to remember that you are in the role of the person who is making the client feel good. A big part of your performance is how convincingly you can smile. I tell my stylists, "I don't care if your car needs a new transmission, if your cat is in the hospital, or if you ate a burrito last night that's having its revenge. Just keep smiling!" The time you are spending with your client is wholly and exclusively about your client's needs, not yours.

◎ *Always, always, always* introduce yourself! Sometimes I'll see a stylist who just walks out and says, "Come back with me, please." Leaving out the crucial part of "Hi, I'm Brenda" or "Hi. I'm Steve" or whatever. That is so inexcusably rude. It's your job as well to make sure that everyone your client comes into contact with, whether it be the receptionist, the shampoo person, or whoever, does the same.

◎ With a new client, I always factor in a few minutes at the start of the appointment to do a quick tour of the salon. I introduce the client to the receptionist and anyone else he meets along the way. It's my little "new client orientation" and it makes a person feel comfortable very quickly.

- I always offer a beverage. I think the offer of a coffee or spring water is the kind of gracious touch that people appreciate and remember.

The Consultation

The consultation is the centerpiece of the stylist-client communication. Obviously, the consultation has a very specific and focused purpose. The aim is to make sure that you and the client are on the same page regarding the service.

- I know stylists who skip the consultation altogether, or else just do it the first time they meet with a client. I think that's a big mistake. Every time I see a client, I factor a consultation aspect into the visit.

- If your salon does not have enough space to devote an entire room to consultations, go to management and request that some kind of area is carved out for this purpose. It's got to be big enough for you and the client to sit together comfortably, and quiet enough so you can hear each other and concentrate on what's being said. If management doesn't want to hear about this, start looking for a job elsewhere because you're in a dead-end shop.

- As a manager, I make sure that the consultation area is equipped with style books, hair color swatches, and a mannequin. You cannot expect to do a proper consultation without these.

◎ This may seem obvious but it's important: make sure that the consultation area is neat and tidied up before you take a client there. A messy consultation area is like a bedroom with an unmade bed; it does not make a good impression. Also, check to make sure that the style books and magazines are in good condition.

◎ Make sure that your client is relaxed and comfortable when you begin the consultation. If that means fetching your client a cup of coffee to start, then do it.

◎ During the consultation and when reviewing the consultation card, keep your judgments to yourself. If the client says she colors, perms, or straightens her own hair, don't act like you've never heard of such a thing. The purpose of the consultation is to gather information. You can use your art of gentle persuasion later on to convince her to let you or someone else in the salon perform these services for her, but first you need to develop an atmosphere of communication and trust.

◎ A big part of the consultation is getting a good hair history. You might have a style you're dying to try on your client, something you think is going to be a revelation. But if you find out in the course of the consultation that the client has never spent more than five minutes a day tending to her hair and the style you're

proposing requires significantly more maintenance, then you're just going to have to go
back to the drawing board.

◎ Shocking as this may sound, there are stylists
out there who don't know what you need to
have on hand in order to do a consultation. You
need a variety of styling books—one for short
hair, one for medium-length, one for long
hair—and photos that show the whole range of
color options. Then, of course, you'll want to
have hair swatches on hand. And don't forget a
portfolio of your own work, if possible. That
means getting photos of your work done.
Simple Polaroids may have to do at first. As
you show the photos, explain why you did
what you did. This way, the new client will develop an understanding of how you work.

◎ Put the time in! Don't rush the consultation
process. People come in with set ideas in their
heads and if you want to "unset" them, you have
to plan on having some extended conversation.
For instance, the client may come in raving about
some haircut that her sister-in-law got and
you're going to have to take the time to take her
through the process, step by step, explaining
why a cut that might look good on her sister-in-
law would not necessarily look good on her.

◎ We've had some talented stylists in our salon
who know how to give a great cut technically,

but who have very little understanding of how a cut works with a client's total look. Part of the consultation should be an observation of and an inquiry into that total look. Does the client favor a classic look with tailored outfits and relatively conservative colors, or is she more drawn to whatever is trendy and hip? You also have to take into account the client's lifestyle. If she's a mom with two little kids under the age of five, don't propose a style that's going to require any sort of real maintenance.

◉ It's important to understand the "dance" that goes on in the consultation. You have to lead. You have to take control of the situation. That means picking up on cues and clues from the client. You need to carefully watch her gestures and facial expressions during the conversation. Is she at ease or is she ill at ease? If she wants to go blonde, does she think it will make her look younger? Read her face and her body language when she answers. And don't forget reflective listening. Give her back what she gave you so you know you're both on the same page.

◉ Don't even think about doing a consultation without having a mirror handy. Even if it has to be a hand-held one, you're going to need it. When both of you look into the mirror together, you'll discover the things you see in common and the things you see that reflect the differences in your perceptions.

- One thing that is really important to learn is never to promise the moon. If a client brings in a picture of an actress and she looks nothing like that actress, then don't pretend you're going to turn her into one of the world's most beautiful women within the hour. You can point out ways in which she can emulate that person—the length of the hair, let's say—but in a tactful and discreet way, you're going to have to provide her with something of a reality test too.

- Maybe this goes without saying, but you've got to be scrupulous about recording relevant information on the consultation card. [Note: See Chapter 6, "Developing Systems," for tips on consultation cards.]

- While you are going through hair style books and discussing your client's particular needs, take this quiet moment to direct her attention to other services available at the salon. Let her know that, in addition to a new haircut, she might also want to consider some of the salon's offerings in the areas of skin and nail care. Use the photos in the styling books to offer examples of these services. If you really want to succeed in this business, economically if in no other way, ticket upgrading has to always be in the back (or maybe even in the front) of your mind.

Handling Client Problems

There's a law of nature that whatever can go wrong does go wrong. Some days at the salon, nothing could feel truer. You will have clients who arrive late and you may have dissatisfied clients. This section will hopefully give you some good, sound advice on what to do in each of these cases.

Tardy Clients

◎ Clients who come late can not only ruin your day, but also can wreak havoc on the schedules of your other clients who may be inclined to hold you responsible for their inconvenience. The first line of defense against tardy clients is to be well acquainted with your salon's lateness policy. I've found that the rule in most salons is that if a client is more than fifteen minutes late, it's time to reschedule. I think that's entirely fair.

◎ Some clients will freak out when you ask them to reschedule. Keep your cool. Explain as calmly and rationally as you can that you have other clients to service and you have to fulfill those responsibilities now. Explain that you also find rushing unacceptable, and that you cannot perform the kind of service you feel capable of under such conditions. If a client decides to take his business elsewhere as a result, so be it. Believe me, it wasn't going to be a great relationship anyway.

◉ If a client shows up late and you can actually take him (let's say you had a cancellation in the following slot), don't let him off the hook so easily. If he does it once and gets off scot-free, he'll do it again. Instead, say something like, "Lucky you! My next appointment isn't for another two hours, so even though you're twenty minutes late, I can take you." This telegraphs the message that lateness is not acceptable under normal circumstances, but in this case, you have decided to accommodate him.

◉ Some people are good clients who just happen to be habitually late. With a client like that, I always schedule her for the last appointment of the day.

◉ If I have a client who tends to run late, I always schedule him a half-hour before he actually has to get there. In other words, if I need him to fill the 3:00 slot, I schedule him for 2:30. Inevitably, he comes at 3:00 and no one's the worse for it.

◉ Clients aren't the only ones who run late. I do, too, at times. When this happens to me, I call my clients to warn them in advance. I get all of my clients' telephone numbers—at home, at work, or their mobiles—and I call them and give them the opportunity to reschedule or to come in a little later. In the event that I can't reach them, I'll go out to meet them when they arrive at the salon, apologize profusely, get them a coffee or mineral water, and maybe even slip in some free product at the end. Even if it costs me out of my own pocket, it's worth it in the long run. Most people will make allowances and will respond well to your efforts to appease them.

Scheduling Mix-Ups

We all make mistakes. Here's how one stylist makes amends:

◉ If you get into a scheduling mix-up, don't make an argument out of whose fault it is. It just happened, that's all. The client is always right. You be the big one and assume all the blame. Believe me, you'll be glad you did. Just say, "I'm sorry. I mixed up the appointment time. Can I reschedule you?" Usually, when you throw yourself on somebody's mercy, they'll respond mercifully.

Handling Unhappy Clients

There is no stylist who has not had the experience of having to deal with an unhappy, dissatisfied, and occasionally very vocal customer. It just comes with the territory. It helps, however, in dealing with the situation to keep a clear goal in mind, and that goal is to make the client happy enough to pay for the service and to come back for more.

- The first order of business is to try to find out why the client is so unhappy. The way to do this is by asking specific questions. Not "Do you like it?" or "Don't you like it?" but "What do you like?" For example, "Are you happy with the length of the bangs?" "Does the length at the nape of the neck work for you?" "Would you like me to take off more around the ears?" It's a game of hot and cold. Your questions should let you know when and if you get warm.

- By all means, if the customer wants something changed and you can change it, go for it! For instance, if she hates the color, look at your book and check the earliest time that you can schedule an appointment to undo what you've done. If you're full up, you'll have to explain to her that you will need to enlist the help of another stylist to fix what she's unhappy with. This isn't going to be music to her ears, but she'll have to understand that this is the way it's done.

- Sometimes, what is done cannot be undone. This is a hard truth about life. If you've cut the hair too short, you can't make it grow back instantly. If this is the case, you will have to take the bull by the horns, admit the truth, offer any options that might help the matter like conditioning treatments or other styling options, and let the chips fall where they may. Maybe your honesty will assuage the client or maybe she'll never come back again. You'll find out soon enough.

- I used to work next to this guy who, when he had an unhappy client, would just keep telling her how great she looked. "Are you crazy? It's fabulous on you! Fabulous!" Guess how many unhappy clients he managed to convince?

- Okay. Here comes the nightmare. You're young, you're inexperienced, and you've messed up royally. Maybe you've cut all wrong around the ears; maybe your color came out orange. And you don't know what to do. Don't tough it out. Go to a more experienced stylist or to your manager for help. This can be done subtly; the client will never have to know. Certainly, in the case of color mishaps, corrections can be done without the client ever being made aware of the problem.

- Sometimes, you just can't win. Your client is unhappy and nothing you say can calm him down. Maybe he's not an easy person to calm down in the first place. This is the time to seek help from your manager. It won't reflect poorly on you; it just might be time for another person to intercede.

◉ Try to schedule a few minutes with your manager after you've been through an experience with an unhappy client. If the manager is any good at managing, you won't walk away feeling worse. It will be a growth opportunity and a good chance to examine the experience from all angles.

◉ I think it's possible to take the "customer is always right attitude" a little too far. I've worked in salons where every time a client opens her mouth with a complaint, it's like you have to have a summit meeting. A lot of those clients think that if they complain, they're going to get a freebie of some sort. I think a salon policy on the issue of complaints is strongly advised.

◉ Our salon has a "three times, you're out" policy. In other words, if a client complains three times about the same person or three times about three different people, we say "Bye-Bye." Life is too short. Three attempts to please a person is all we can afford. Keep in mind that there are some people who can never be pleased, no matter how hard you try.

◉ We regularly do client surveys in our salon. We offer the clients a 20 percent coupon on retail if they fill out a survey. You can learn a lot about keeping customers happy from a good survey.

Getting and Keeping Clients

In order to be a successful cosmetologist, you have to have a really solid client base. Here are some thoughts on how to go about developing that.

- I suppose nothing could be more obvious than this, but I think the foundation to a strong client base lies in providing good service. Don't expect to rush through your work and have the customer come back to you. It isn't going to happen.

- To me, it's all about trust. Your client should be able to trust that you're not going to keep him waiting (except perhaps in case of an emergency). He should be able to trust you to give him the haircut he asks for (after you've had your consultation). And a relationship based on trust means that you don't try to retail to the client any products that you can't personally recommend. Without the trust, the relationship is not going to last.

- Maintain your professional standards at all times. That means no idle gossip and no invasion of your client's privacy. What's more, you will not allow the client to invade your privacy.

- Look your best. Carry yourself well. You have an image to project. Don't forget that.

- I've known stylists who have this weird idea that the more time they spend performing services on their clients, the more the client will feel that the service was worthwhile. I think that's a lot of hogwash. Most people are more than happy to spend less rather than more time in the salon, as long as the service is first-rate. So pick up your speed, ladies and gentlemen.

- Don't worry about being corny. Clients love to get birthday cards. Record your client's birthdate on the consultation card and send a birthday card out well in advance, maybe with a special offer or a coupon.

- In one salon where I worked, they had this great idea that I've carried with me wherever I've gone. It's a kind of dual business card. Half the card has your information on it and the other half is for your client's name and contact information. If the client likes your work, ask her to give the card out to friends and associates, signing her name to it. Everyone who comes to you that way means a 10 percent reduction in the next service for your client.

- I've found that an excellent way to build up a client base is by partnering up with other local businesses. Florists, for instance, are always doing weddings, and what is another service that people who are getting married look for? Hairstyling, of course! So try a card swap with a florist, a bridal salon, a clothing store, and so on.

◉ I happen to feel comfortable with public speaking (I know not everyone is), but I make it a point, a few times a year, to speak to a local women's group or a PTA or a chamber of commerce. I put together a short program, maybe 20 minutes, on image. A "Dress for Success" kind of thing, with tips on makeup, hair, skin care, and so on. I always bring business cards with me and I've gotten a lot of clients that way.

◉ Once you've got a client, it's important to "glue" her to you with some aggressive rebooking. Rebooking is just another form of selling, except that instead of selling conditioner or some other retail product, you're selling yourself.

◉ The best time to think about getting your client back into the salon is while he is still in the chair. And the best way to encourage your client to book another appointment before he leaves is to simply talk with him, ask questions, and listen carefully to his answers.

◉ Knowing your client and having an ongoing conversation with her will furnish you with openings to bring up the subject of rebooking. For instance, you might say something like,

"Boy, that vacation in Hawaii sounds amazing. But you want to be careful how you handle your hair now, after having been in the sun for two weeks. It would be a good idea to do a couple of deep conditioning treatments before we do color again. Since you usually color every two months, why don't we book a couple of those treatments this month?"

◉ Keep an ear out for any big days coming up for your client, whether they are weddings, parties, job interviews, class reunions, or whatever, and utilize these events as opportunities to suggest rebookings. Your client will not chafe at the idea. In fact, she'll be grateful that you're thinking about her.

 . . . And a Few Special Cases

◉ One area of potential conflict between you and a client can arise around the client's children if she brings them to the salon with her. I've managed three salons and I've found that the match of children and salons just doesn't work. I love children, but the only salon that a child should be in is a salon for children. One of those places that has motorcycles to sit in or big shoes or jungle gyms or whatever. A real kid environment.

- At our salon, we instituted a "no children" policy, just as we have a "no smoking" policy, and we stand by it. Now that might make us sound like terrible people, but guess what? Our business has picked up! The clients who come to us want peace and quiet during this experience, and it's their money. They should have what they want.

- We don't have a "no children" policy, but we certainly don't make the salon kid-friendly. For one thing, we don't offer any children's discounts, so that discourages some customers right off the bat.

- How best to handle having family and friends as a client is a situation that comes up for a lot of stylists. I personally do my family for free, because in my book, family is family. For most other people who have any kind of personal connection to me, I do an exchange of services. I cut my bookkeeper's hair; she keeps my books. I cut my dog groomer's hair; she grooms my dog. You get the idea.

- Everybody's different about family and friends because we all have different types of relationships. I'm pretty hard-headed about it. I work really hard to make my living and my designated work hours are precious to me. Those are the hours that I can make income. If family wants to come to me during my designated work hours, than they have to pay my full fee. If they come after hours, I do them for free, just charging for the price of whatever product is needed. I think that's fair, don't you?

◉ You'd be amazed, but when you get into this line of work, suddenly you'll encounter family you never knew you had. Third cousins thrice removed! You've got to draw a line somewhere. Don't be shy about it.

Handling Client Health Problems

Some stylists have a hard time knowing what to do when a client with a health problem appears in the salon. Here are a couple of ideas:

◉ Honesty is the best policy in a situation like this. If there is a scalp condition other than simple dandruff for which you can recommend a dandruff shampoo, I would recommend that the client see a dermatologist immediately. Do not bring the problem to the attention to others in the salon. You don't want to embarrass your client. If the problem is head lice, send the client to the drug store to speak with a pharmacist. Then clean every brush and comb in the place!

◉ Address the problem in private. Don't just turn the client away; make sure he understands that something like head lice is not at all uncommon and that it is eminently treatable. You can inform the client about special shampoos, the necessity to clean bed clothes and sheets, and the need to see a doctor for extreme cases. Make the client feel as comfortable as possible. This is not an easy experience for the client and you want him to return after the problem is resolved.

If the problem is discovered during consultation, the stylist should:

- give the client the benefit of the doubt by asking if he's noticed any prior problems with his scalp.

- remove the risk of client embarrassment or the risk of alarming the client by telling him first that the problem is very fixable.

- make a professional opinion that he should not be servicing the client until the problem is taken care of.

- not attempt to diagnose the problem, but instead of outright refusing to do the client's hair, causing more embarrassment, recommend that the client does not have his hair done at that time, as it may be harmful to his condition.

- reschedule the client's appointment to let the client know he'd be happy to service the client in the future.

Chapter 10

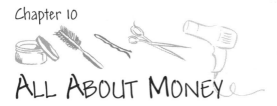

ALL ABOUT MONEY

M oney.

Ah, now there's a topic to get the juices flowing.

There is considerable money to be made in the cosmetology field, and, in fact, you may already be making it. If so, that's good news for you. On the other hand, if you're not yet where you'd like to be, don't despair. Keep at it and chances are your efforts will pay off financially. In any event, in this chapter we are offering an elementary overview designed to get you into a thinking mode on the subject of money. As a cosmetologist, surely you know that the importance of continuing education. A cosmetologist needs to stay on top of the ever-changing fashions and techno-logical advances in the field. Just so, all of us need to engage in continuing education when it comes to the subject of how to manage our money. So, while this overview may serve as a nice way to open up the discussion, its purpose is really to inspire you to do more reading and research on your own.

 ## The Psychology of Money

Money carries an extraordinary emotional charge in the lives of many, if not most, people. As we grow up, we are given all kinds of different messages from our families on the subject of money.

Money makes the world go around.

Money is the root of all evil.

Marry a rich man.

Get a regular paycheck.

Never tell anybody what you make.

We have to process all these messages and come up with something that we feel comfortable living by.

◉ In my family, the worst thing in the world you could do was talk about money. To me, it made money into this incredible unknowable thing, and it's taken me a good part of my adult life to realize that money is just a tool. If you know how to use it, you can get things done. It's not a mystery. It's a reality.

◉ I come from a very old-fashioned family where it was felt that money was something that men dealt with, not women. Throughout my marriage, I lived by that credo. Then my husband left me and suddenly I had a whole lot of money-learning to do.

◉ My brother-in-law, who's one of those dot-com geniuses, tells me that money is a game. His point is not that it isn't real or that you should convince yourself that what you're using is play money, but, more to the point, that you should have some fun with money. No matter what you earn, you should use some portion of it, even a tiny bit, to grow in an exciting way.

◉ It's hard not to care about money when you live in the United States. I grew up in The Philippines and it was a whole different story there. In the United States, we have a consumer culture. Beautiful things are advertised all the time, and people are throwing credit cards at you so that you can buy those beautiful things. You've got to be careful about caring too much about material goods at the expense of what is nonmaterial, like nature and love and spirituality.

◎ When you live in a society as affluent as ours, where the net worth of the rich is measured not in millions but in billions, you run the risk of equating material worth with inner worth. The more money you have, the better or more successful you believe you are as a person. But money and stuff are one thing; the real value of a person is quite another. The most successful human being I ever knew was my father, a housepainter. Why? Because he loved people and people loved him.

◎ When it comes to money, you have to strike a balance that you're comfortable with. How much of your life are you willing to dedicate to making money? How much time away from your personal life do you feel you can afford? I remember once reading about this man who resigned as the CEO of a large company so he would have more time for his private life. He said, "I never heard of anybody saying at the end of their life that they regretted the time they spent with their family."

◎ Be in control of your money: it's yours. That doesn't mean, obviously, that you have to manage it on your own. But if you're going to use a financial advisor, which I think most of us can benefit by, you have to make sure they're highly recommended by people you trust, and that they speak to you in a way that is totally accessible and without jargon. If they can't do that, then look for someone else. Don't let yourself be intimidated by money. After all, you're the one who made it!

The Financial Pyramid

No doubt you've seen the Food Guide Pyramid at some point in your life. You may have studied it in health class with grains at the bottom, fruit and vegetables on the next layer, dairy and meat, fish, poultry, eggs, dry beans, and nuts above that, and at the narrow peak, fats, oils, and sweets to be used sparingly. Well, there's also such a thing as a Financial Pyramid, which offers a graphic representation of your lifetime financial goals. At the base are your Values and Goals: do you want to retire at 45? Become a philanthropist? Live in a camper? Figure it out and make your base. The next step shows your basic living expenses: food, shelter, clothing, transportation, and the like. Before you go on to spend money on other things, you have to meet those needs. Once you've budgeted for basics, you can climb up to your layer of Savings, Credit, and Insurance. From there, you might move on to Owning a Home. At the summit is Investing for the Future, which addresses your childrens' college tuitions, your retirement, and so on. The Financial Pyramid helps you prioritize your goals and allot your resources.

Budgeting

Some people balk at the idea of budgeting. They regard it as an kind of activity that certain people might want to bother with, as certain people enjoy burdensome tasks like ironing or polishing shoes, but it's not something that they need to do. The reality, however, is that we all need to budget. Even people making enormous sums of money need to budget. There is no shortage of tragic tales about people who made scads of money but lived so high on the hog that nothing was left at the end of their run. Let's have a look at what your colleagues have to say on the subject of budgeting.

- Most people think of budgeting as a matter of dollars and cents: what comes in and what goes out. But budgeting is more than that. The real value of budgeting is that it helps you focus on your goals. You see exactly what you need to do and how long it will take to get you where you want to be. For instance, if you have $100 a month left over after your expenses, you might want to save $80 of that money each month and put $20 a month toward the sound system you want to buy. In a certain amount of time, you will have saved enough money to buy that system, which is different than just putting the purchase on a credit card and then paying it off at 23 percent.

◎ Whenever I mentor young people coming into this field, I always start early talking to them about budgeting. With many of them, I have to start with the fundamentals by defining what income and expenses are. Some people think of income only as salary, but it's more than that. It could be an allowance from your parents or spouse, or alimony or child support payments or welfare payments or food stamps. It could include student financial aid and tax refunds. Gifts are income. If your uncle gives you $100 at Christmas, that's income. Interest earned on savings is income too, as are dividends earned on investments.

◎ It's important to get down certain basic terminology right at the outset: like the difference between gross and net. The total amount of your income, collected from all your various sources, is your gross income. If you're working, your employer withholds certain amounts from your paycheck in order to pay federal and local taxes, social security (FICA), group insurance premiums, union dues, pension contributions, and other deductions. The amount of money left over is called your net income, which is, of course, less than your gross income.

◎ When you're budgeting, you have to know the difference between fixed and variable expenses. Fixed expenses don't change. Your rent or mortgage payments, your utilities, telephone, car payments, insurance payments; these are all fixed expenses. Variable expenses are those that come up now and then and are unpredictable. You bite down on an olive pit and break a tooth. You've got a variable expense. Your transmission goes; variable. Get it?

◎ A wise person, my Uncle Max, once told me, when I was starting out in life, to keep in mind "the Four A's of Budgeting." You *account* for your income and expenses. You *analyze* the situation after you've had a look at the numbers. You *allocate* your income, using it as you see fit. You *adjust* your budget as necessary.

◎ The way to start budgeting is to keep track of everything you spend money on for at least a couple of months. Carry around a little note pad with you and jot down all your expenses such as cabs, lunch, magazines, an ice cream cone, and a double mocha latté. Whenever you spend money, jot it down, with the date, and don't forget to enter those purchases you make by credit card or over the Internet. They didn't come free, you know. The idea is to step back after a couple of months and to look at your patterns. You'll get a sense of where the money has flowed, and if it needs to be redirected, then you can start to do that.

◎ Once you've gotten a firm grip on how and where you've been spending your money, you can run your tallies and come to some initial conclusions. The first thing you'll be looking at is whether your expenses exceeded your income, which obviously is not a good thing. Were you able to cover all your fixed expenses? Did any sudden big expenses come up? Did you pay off your credit card balance? If not, did you make the minimum payment? These are hard questions, and a lot of people procrastinate about asking them, but the longer you wait to do this work, the bigger the hole you're liable to dig for yourself.

◎ Try not to panic when you're engaged in the work of budgeting. It is scary sometimes, but few problems are insurmountable, thank goodness. The first thing you have to do is look at your fixed expenses and make sure you have the money for them. Then you can look at your variable expenses and start chopping away. Cigarettes? Now there's a no-brainer. They cost you a fortune plus they give you lung cancer. Instead of premium "designer" coffees bought at a high-priced chain, scale down to a regular good cup of coffee like the ones that people used to drink. Buy your clothes at the end of the season when prices are slashed. Walk if possible instead of using public transportation. The health benefits are as good as the money-saving benefits.

◎ I always advise young people starting out to factor an emergency fund into their budget. Your car breaks down and suddenly you need $300 to replace the alternator. You can borrow from your parents, if you're lucky, or you could have budgeted in an emergency fund, channeling some of the money into it that you might otherwise have used for impulse buys.

◎ It's good and rewarding to have long-term goals that you save for like a vacation or a new coat or a piece of furniture. These things are expensive, and saving for them over a period of months creates a kind of financial discipline that will serve you well as time goes on.

◎ Budgets need to be reviewed regularly and changed as necessary. A raise means a change in your budget. A layoff means a change in your budget. A baby means a change in your budget. When times are good, you will want to treat yourself to some goodies (again, of course, those that are within that budget). When times are not so good, you have to tighten your belt.

Savings and Credit

Young Americans today are saving less than the generations that came before them and are running up higher credit card debts. This situation needs to be looked at and corrected.

◉ My great-great-grandmother, who grew up in a mining camp in Montana, hid all her money in a tin can that she kept underneath a pot belly stove. Now that's living dangerously. Today, we have reliable financial institutions in which to save our money. When choosing a home for your savings, you have to ask questions to make sure you're getting what you want. Up to what amount are your deposits insured and by whom (federal insurance such as FDIC is a better risk than state insurance funds). What are the interest rates? How easily can you get to your money? What types of accounts are offered?

◉ There are a lot of different types of saving accounts. I tell most of the young people I work with to consider the basic four: a passbook account which you can open with very little money but that pays very little interest; a money market account with interest rates that fluctuate with the market rate, but which require a minimum balance and which often restrict withdrawals; a certificate of deposit (CD) which offers the highest rates but ties up your money for a lengthy period of time; and an individual retirement account (IRA) that is used to put aside money for retirement and which carries strict penalties regarding premature withdrawal of funds.

◎ You'll see that the more income you earn, the more types of savings account you'll need. If you're unsure about which direction to go, check with a friend or family member you trust, or schedule a meeting with a customer service representative at a bank. That's what they're there for.

◎ I know people who never ever use credit cards and I know people who use credit cards every time they turn around. As far as I'm concerned, there's a middle ground. Your job is to see if you can find it.

◎ Some people just don't understand credit. They think it's there as some kind of public service so you can buy those leather pants you're dying to have without having to bother to wait until you save up the money for them. What some people don't seem to realize is that anything you buy on credit will cost you more than if you paid cash for that item. You have to consider your interest charges.

◎ Maybe you grew up hearing how buying on credit is a terrible thing. If you still think it is, by all means stay away from it. On the other hand, credit can work well for you. If you need snow tires to get you through the winter and don't have the money for them right now but think you can pay it off over a period of some months, go for it. Same with a medical expense or some other necessity. That's different, however, from using credit cards to buy a new ski outfit or a cashmere sweater. Succumbing to impulse buys is what gets you into trouble with credit cards.

◎ Playing the catch-up game around credit is exhausting and you really wind up the loser. If you accumulate a large balance and all you ever do is make the minimum monthly payment, then all you're doing is paying off interest without ever reducing the sum you've borrowed.

◎ Be very careful about your credit rating. If you don't pay your bills, particularly your credit card bills, your credit rating will take a nosedive and you will be unable to secure a mortgage or a business loan, and may close off other important avenues as well.

◎ All credit cards are not created equal. When you've made the decision that you want a credit card, you need to shop around to make sure you get one that has advantageous features. Most important is the annual percentage rate (APR), which is the interest you will be charged per year on the amount you finance. Some cards have astronomical APRs, up to 23 percent, which, in this climate where credit card companies are competing with each other for consumers, is ridiculous. You also have to pay attention to the microscopic print that details the finance charges. These explain the interest, fees, service charges, insurance, and other variables, and they differ from one company to the next.

◉ Some people don't realize that there's a difference between a credit card that you can pay off over time, and a charge card that you have to pay off in full each month.

◉ Getting credit in the first place can be a challenge. I remember when I first applied for a loan, I was refused because I had no credit record. So how do you develop a credit record, I wondered, if no one wants to give you credit? It's a Catch-22, right? My boyfriend suggested I take out a small installment loan—at that time we needed a new fridge—and he would co-sign the loan because he had a good credit history. As I paid off the loan for a fridge, I developed a credit history, too.

◉ Signing up for utilities in your own name, even though the deposit can be hefty, is another good way to start up a credit history.

- You should know, if anyone ever questions your credit rating, that you have a right to see your credit record. Credit records are maintained by credit bureaus, and they can and do make mistakes. When I went to refinance my mortgage, it was almost denied to me because a credit bureau reported that I had defaulted on mortgage payments. Of course, it turned out to be a different person with the same name but if I hadn't checked, it would still be following me around. For a nominal fee, you can see your credit record and can know who else has seen it in the past six months. If any of the information on it is incorrect, you can have it checked out and changed, with corrected copies sent to anyone who has seen the incorrect report.

 Debt

Debt is not a pleasant situation to be in, although a great many Americans live with it from year to year.

- A lot of debt goes unnamed. For instance, there are some people who carry huge credit card debts but they act like that's not really in debt. They're fooling themselves, and while they're doing it, they're getting in deeper and deeper.

- Debt comes with certain telltale signs you should pay attention to. Do you pay only the minimum on your credit cards each month? Do you juggle bills, skipping some to pay others? Are you gripped by panic every time an unexpected major expense comes up like a major car repair? Do you moonlight or depend on overtime to make ends meet? Do you borrow from family or friends? If these scenarios sound familiar, you don't have to feel terrible—believe me, you're not alone—but you will want to do something to gain some control over the situation.

◎ Some of the younger stylists have confided in me their fears about their debt, and I tell them I've been there. Here's what you have to do, I say. Start by going back to your budget and see where you can find places to cut expenses. Okay, maybe you'll have to do without that expensive eyeliner for a while until you pay off some of this debt, but you can live with that. Then I tell them to call up the credit card companies or any of their other creditors and work out a schedule for paying off the debt. Another thing you can do is consolidation: putting all your debt under one roof and working out a real plan to take care of it. If you ask around, you'll be sure to find out about reputable credit consolidation companies that can help you organize your debt payoff.

◎ If you're seriously in debt, get serious about resolving the problem. Contact an organization whose express purpose is to help people get out of debt. American Consumer Credit Counseling and the National Foundation for Consumer Credit are two such organizations that provide credit counseling services, either free or for a very small fee.

Mortgages

Mortgages are a form of debt, but they can work positively in your behalf in the sense that they can offer significant tax benefits.

◉ If you're buying a house, check out interest-only mortgages. These are completely tax deductible for the first ten years of the mortgage. In other words, you'll be able to write off your complete monthly payment. Plus, if you pre-pay the principle at any point, you'll not only lower your monthly payment but also you'll shorten the mortgage period. This is in contrast to a fixed mortgage where the payment remains the same and you just shorten the period.

◉ The thing you've got to be careful about with the interest-only mortgages is that it's only interest-free for the first 10 years. After that, it turns into a 15-year amortized mortgage.

◉ Keep in mind that a low monthly mortgage payment can free up money for investments in the stock market or wherever. Or you might decide to put some of the extra money into home improvements, increasing the value of your property, and, in turn, increasing your equity.

 Investing

Down the road a bit, you may find yourself with some extra money to grow. One thing you might decide to do is invest it in the stock market.

◉ One thing we've all learned from the dot-com experience is that prudence should always be a part of how your approach the market. When you buy a stock, it should be the result of careful research. Your research. You should closely examine a stock's twelve-month price history, and its profits and earnings ratio before buying.

◉ Every stock has a high and a low. When you buy a stock, you need to know whether you're buying high or selling low.

◉ My financial advisor told me that as an investor, I shouldn't be buying and selling all the time. That's what traders do. As an investor, I should set up a long-term portfolio that takes into account my goals and my risk tolerance, and I shouldn't let day-to-day fluctuations affect my long-term time frame.

- One lesson I was taught by my cousin, who's a stockbroker, is that most people sell the stocks that are going up without thinking about its continued growth over the long run, and hold on to the ones that aren't going down, thinking they'll do better. He told me it should be the other way around.

- I've done well in the market and one reason is because I was well taught. My boyfriend, who's in the financial community, taught me how important it is to study the fundamentals of a company before you buy into it. You have to look at the management, at whether the company dominates the market, if they're in the #1, #2, or #3 position, and what kind of investment they make in research and development (R & D), which is how they're preparing for the future. If you do this research and things come up looking good, it's unlikely you'll go too wrong. At least, I haven't so far, knock wood.

- The best thing I ever did for my financial picture was to join an investment club. There are eight of us and we've pooled money to hire an advisor who consults with us occasionally. We're doing great!

- The key to investing, as far as I'm concerned, is diversification. Never, ever, put all your eggs in one basket.

- It's up to each individual investor to determine the level of risk that he is comfortable with. Your stockbroker can't determine that for you. You have to figure it out for yourself and then strike a comfortable balance in your portfolio.

- Personally, I look into more defensive types of securities and I encourage others to do the same. I buy utilities, food groups, and basic companies that are always going to be there, in good times and bad. That's just my philosophy.

- We've had the era of trendy stocks. Remember all the dot.coms? Now I'm looking at tax-free municipal bonds. Okay, highway construction may not be all that exciting, but investing in these municipal bonds is a relatively safe bet these days. At the very least, they can help diversify an otherwise risky portfolio and you'll save money at tax time, since the interest is free from federal, state, and local taxes.

Retirement and Other Long-Term Savings Goals

People are living longer than they ever have, which means we have to prepare for the future more than ever. The future of our children is also something that needs to be taken into account.

- My financial advisor told me that to ensure that you are saving enough for retirement, whether it's in an IRA or outside of an IRA, you need to look at what your current cash flow needs are. You then add 3.1 percent to that annually until the point of retirement. This will give you the dollar figure you need after taxes.

- Retirement planning means planning for the unknown. That's hard to do. One thing you know for sure is that you don't want to outlive your money. That means it's important to remove as much nondeductible debt as possible—such as credit card interest—while you're still working. Any remaining tax-deductible debt such as that from the interest on a mortgage may actually be beneficial in that it can put you into a lower tax bracket during your retirement phase.

- In a traditional IRA, contributions of up to $2,000 a year can be made. Under certain income limits, the contribution can be tax deductible.

- In 1998, Congress created the Roth IRA and this has been a boon for a lot of people. With the Roth, you can contribute up to $2,000 a year within certain income guidelines, and if you've held it over five years, everything is tax-free forever. Also, if you continue to work after you're 70 and a half years old, you can continue to make contributions to your Roth IRA, which you can't do with a traditional IRA. Check into this with your financial advisor. It may be just the right answer for you.

◉ Your best bet is to take part in your company's 401(k) plan. A lot of people never bother to sign up, which is a huge mistake. These plans allow employees to contribute up to $10,500 pre-tax dollars per year. A lot of companies even match employees' contributions. The money is invested in tax-deferred accounts until your retirement. It comes out to be a real bundle.

◉ I've got an IRA brokerage account that allows me to do everything under one roof. The brokerage house lets you do the money markets, the CDs, stocks, bonds, everything and anything you're looking for. That means you can do without having four or five different accounts for your different modes of investing. Also, the restrictions that limit how an IRA can be invested don't exist within a brokerage account, since any publicly traded investment can be placed in the account and can grow tax-deferred.

◉ One question I've had over the years when I've changed jobs is what do I do with my 401(k)? The answer I've always been given is to move it with my job. I put it into an IRA rollover account where I can invest in mutual funds, stocks, and bonds. There are no costs or penalties because I'm keeping it in a retirement fund.

◉ One thing nobody ever tells you is that you can save too much for retirement and have negative tax consequences as a result. One way of getting around that is by taking occasional distributions that will be taxed as ordinary income. You can also just roll your IRA into your estate. The down side will be that your heirs will receive their inheritance after estate taxes and ordinary income taxes are paid. That could be as much as 75 percent of the estate. So if you want to avoid that, you really should consult with an estate planner.

◉ You can't start too early with investments for your kids. The first thing to do for your baby with regard to money is to file for a Social Security number. Then think about the investment vehicle you're going to use. With the long time horizon a baby has, you can afford to have a little more risk in the portfolio.

◉ I went the route of zero-coupon bonds for my kid's college tuition. These are fixed income investments that pay no periodic interest. They're just there because at the end of the run, you know exactly how much you're going to get. There's no risk. There's no guesswork. In X years, you'll have X dollars. Because of the way they're set up, they're often sold at a discount, so shop around (or have your personal shopper do the shopping). And, in most cases, the interest is tax-free.

This has been something of a whirlwind tour through the subject of money. It's the barest of beginnings. It's up to you to keep learning. The more you learn, the better you should be able to do with your investments and with finances in general.

Chapter 11

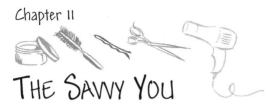

THE SAVVY YOU

Speaking of survival—for that, after all, is the word that features in the title of this book—we should all recognize that at this point in the 21st century, if we are to survive in today's work world, we need to be flexible, forward-thinking, and proactive about our careers. Resting on our laurels is not an option. No matter how long you've been out in the workforce or how many years of service you've put into a particular job, if the fit no longer feels right, then it is time to consider change. Inertia, which means going nowhere and doing nothing, is totally counter to success.

No matter how many times you've been through the job-hunting search, however, each time seems to have its own set of anxieties attached to it. It is not a fun process, but keep in mind that it can be a highly rewarding process that you can become good at. Like everything else in life, job-hunting relies on a set of skills. When you learn these skills and hone them, you'll always feel empowered to be in control of your own career.

An important aspect of job-hunting has to do with networking: connecting with and listening to other people. Think of this chapter, then, as an exercise in networking. You will be hearing from others in the field who have shared your dreams and your problems, and who have found useful and creative approaches to the job-hunting situation.

Laying the Groundwork

Is the right job out there waiting for you? The only way to find out is for you to start looking. Don't let yourself languish in a work situation where you feel overworked, undervalued, and underpaid. But before you hit the street, do a self-check to see how ready you are.

◉ I encourage everyone I mentor to take a proactive stance when it comes to finding a job. Don't wait for someone to tap you on the shoulder; for most of us, it doesn't usually happen that way. But when you decide to look for a job, that's when you should do a review of yourself. You need to have a good grasp of just how valuable you would be to an employer.

◉ I always want to be sure that I'm working at my full potential before I start looking around to make a change. So what I do is I "grade" myself. I make up a list of criteria—my attitude (is it positive enough?), my appearance (is it professional?), punctuality, continuing education, my teamwork skills—and I really gave some hard thought as to how well I'm doing. If I'm not sure, I'll ask someone I trust to help review me. When I feel that I've gotten my grades up to an "A" level, then I feel ready to look for a job.

◉ It always amazes me how many people stay in dead-end jobs. It's not because that's the easy way out. Usually these jobs have some really serious drawbacks, and there's nothing easy about feeling frustrated and disappointed. I think the reason so many people allow themselves to be undervalued has to do with self-image and motivation. So, in some cases, the job hunt really should begin with a hard look at yourself and maybe even some intervention from a counselor or a psychotherapist if you think your self-esteem and motivation need some major overhauling.

Making the Right Match

There are so many career options available to cosmetologists that making the right choice can be a challenge.

◎ Coming out of beauty school, I guess almost everyone I knew started in a small independent salon. And most of us, of course, started as apprentices. That's just the way it was. The bad news about small independent salons is that there isn't any uniformity or quality control from one to the other, and I've heard plenty of horror stories. The good news is that, if you're lucky, you'll wind up working in an intimate setting with a real human being. There is no better way to start than that.

◎ My choice was to start with an independent salon chain. It had some of the perks of a free-standing independent salon in that there was a certain intimacy and warmth about it, but it also provided the opportunity for growth. I was moved around to two other salons in the chain and I got to try a little bit of everything. I finally wound up in color and probably never would have if I hadn't had the opportunity to experiment.

◎ What nobody tells you about the job search is that *you* have to know what you want! It's not just a matter of money or vacation or insurance plans. There are a lot of indefinable factors that go into your decision. For instance, I've always worked in salon chains. I started with a couple of budget ones and for the last 10 years, I've been working with one of the real blue-chip department store chains. Why was this right for me? Because I discovered things about myself. I never wanted to settle down; that's just my personality. I wanted to be a free agent, living wherever I chose. Working for the chains the way I do, I've been able to live in Miami, Los Angeles, and Honolulu. That's the life I love, but of course that's not the life for everyone.

◎ I own my own salon now, but I loved starting out working for one of the large national chains. I didn't start out with much in the way of support as a youngster, so this gave me a lot of what I needed. I had a secure regular paycheck, benefits, paid training, all the continuing education I wanted, and the chance to build up a clientele on somebody else's coin. I never would have gotten as much in a small independent salon and it was just what I needed to start me out right in life.

◎ I'd like to put in a word for the budget chains. I think they're a great place to start. Okay, the money may not be the best, but you don't have to worry so much about slipping up. Men and kids, who represent a lot of the clientele, are not going to raise a ruckus if you don't do a brilliant cut. And you get to experiment with a lot of different styles. You develop speed and confidence, knowing that you can give a good haircut in 15 minutes so many times throughout the day.

◎ What is so important to remember in this field is that where you start out doesn't in any way determine where you will end up. Now that I'm a so-called seasoned professional, I give over time to beauty schools where I often give talks and even mentor students. One of the messages I continually try to drum into them is that there are so many choices in this field. You could be a color specialist, a nail care or skin care specialist, a platform artist, or an educator. You could specialize in texture services or hair extensions. You could discover this whole other aspect of yourself—let's say you have a genius for selling—and you might become a retail specialist, working in a salon or a spa or a department store. That kind of capacity for communication might lead you to become a product educator down the road.

◎ As a manager, I always keep an eye out for people who have an aptitude for management. Some people enter this field thinking that they are purely creative types, then discover that what they're really good at is solving problems. These people are gold and I search for them.

When I find them, I groom them for bigger and better management positions. I don't let them out of my sight!

◎ I tell young people in the field to think big. If you've got a dream, go after it. You know, a lot of people enter this field because they just love glamour and excitement. Well, there's nothing wrong with loving glamour and excitement, ladies and gentlemen. You're in the right place! So if you're working for a chain and you're not getting the glamour and excitement you dreamed of, do some research and find out what it takes to become a makeup artist for stage and screen or a session hairstylist doing magazine shoots with top models.

◎ As long as you're not willing to get stuck in a rut, there are no boundaries in this field. Your talent and energy can take you to the most extraordinary places. I knew a guy who went to beauty school with me. He worked hard, he kept his eyes and ears open, and he kept on learning. Moving from one job to another, he discovered that he was good at meeting deadlines, at working within a budget, at managing people, and at coming up with creative solutions. He had it all, in other words, and now he's an Artistic Director for a Fortune 500 company, attending to all their esthetic needs. He coordinates their conventions, banquets, and industrial shows. And he started out cutting hair!

- Do the research. Talk to people. You'll find out that there are job directions you never even thought of. Do you like writing? Work on a fashion magazine writing about hair, or for a trade journal or a manufacturer. Do you want a nice pension to retire on? Become a state board examiner. Whatever works for you. But how will you know what works unless you know what's out there?

Regarding Résumés

A good pair of shears is a cosmetologist's basic tool and a good résumé is the basic tool of a cosmetologist in search of a job. The résumé, which is the written summary of your education and work experience, will tell potential employers at a glance all about your achievements and accomplishments. Here are some thoughts from your colleagues on the subject of résumés.

- Rule #1: Keep it short. One page. Nothing more.

- Make sure you put your résumé on good quality paper. Don't go rainbow-crazy. Maybe you think pink is your color or orange is cheerful, but other people might hate the colors pink or orange, so why start out with that strike against you? Stick with white, buff, or gray. You might think that's a little boring, but most people would regard those choices as tasteful and classic.

◉ You might have a great résumé in terms of layout and the accomplishments you're listing, but if you don't have the necessary contact information—address, telephone number, email address—then what good is it going to do you? Make sure that information appears on your cover letter as well.

◉ When it comes to résumés, there's a big argument over how to arrange them. Check with library sources or on the Internet for format. Some people like to arrange the résumé by chronologically listing positions held. Other people like to arrange it by functions performed. You'll have to check it out and decide for yourself.

◉ When listing your accomplishments, be as specific as you can. Take an inventory before you even sit down to do your résumé so that you have a clear view of what it is you've actually accomplished. For instance, ask yourself focused, concrete questions like, "How many clients do I serve weekly?" "What is my service ticket average?" "What is my client retention rate?" "What percent of my clinic revenue comes from retailing?" Once you've done this, you might come up with some impressive statistics that you'll certainly want to use on the résumé.

- Don't forget to list any honors and awards you've gotten, and make sure you include memberships in any professional organizations.

- List all of your continuing education courses.

- Don't forget that people are busy, so make your pitch clear and concise. Don't use long, elaborate sentences. Keep it simple and straightforward.

- If you look at the literature on creating résumés, they'll stress how you should always use "action verbs." You *developed, achieved, created, coordinated, maintained, formulated, introduced,* and so on. These words make you sound like a powerful force, which you may very well be!

- Proofread, my friends, proofread. Misspellings and poor grammar will mean points taken off. And in this competitive job market, you can't afford to lose points on stuff like that. Just ask a friend or family member to give your résumé the once-over. But make sure that person is a decent proofreader. If necessary, go back to your beauty school and draw on resources there for this task.

- Nothing, nothing, nothing goes into the résumé about your salary requirements. Could that be any clearer? Any talk about salary is restricted to your interview, and only if and when the interviewer brings the subject up.

- No photos, please. That makes your résumé look like a most wanted notice you'd find in the post office.

- If nothing else, remember this rule: *never, ever, lie on your résumé.* It will come back to haunt you, and when the grapevine gets hold of what you've done, you might have really serious problems finding a job in the town you live in.

- Some résumé reference sources will tell you to list personal interests like hobbies or the fact that you're a member of the local bird watchers society or whatever. I've never cared for that on a résumé. Frankly, I just don't find it very relevant.

- Don't include personal references on your résumé. It's safe to assume that everyone has someone who can speak well of her. Just list a few professional references. If a specific job asks for personal references on its job application, than that's another story.

Another useful resource to develop for your job search is the employment portfolio. This is a collection, usually bound, of photos and other materials that exhibit your skills and accomplishments in your field. Portfolios may include any and all of the following:

- Diplomas, both high school and cosmetology school.

- Awards and achievements received while a cosmetology student.

- Current résumé, focusing on accomplishments.

- Letters of reference from former employers.

- Summary of continuing education and/or copies of actual training certificates.

- Statement of membership in industry and other professional organizations.

- Statement of relevant civic affiliations and/or community activities.

- Before and after photographs of services you have performed on clients or models.

- A brief statement about why you have chosen a career in cosmetology.

- Any other information that you regard as relevant.

Zeroing In

With your résumé in shape and perhaps a portfolio assembled, you can start to target those establishments where you might like to work. Keep in mind, however, these pointers.

- We all hear a lot about dream jobs. Mostly, it's a bunch of hooey. To me, dream jobs are like dream families: no one I know has one. All jobs come with their problems, and usually the problems are too much or too little work, crazy people, long commutes, no room for advancement, or any and all of the above.

- Let your fingers do the walking through the telephone book. It's a great resource. I find it a lot more "user-friendly" than the Internet, which I think is over-hyped for the purposes of job searches. I do know some people who have found jobs through the net, but most people, including myself, find that it takes a long time to navigate the different sites and this time might be used more effectively otherwise.

- Do we all know by now that relying on "help wanted" ads in the newspaper is probably the least effective way of landing a good job? Many jobs are never advertised and some businesses that do advertise only run these ads because they are required to, when, in fact, what they're really planning to do, is promote from inside.

- Networking is a great way to find a job. It involves contacting people for information. For instance, you might have a cousin who knows someone who has a cousin who works for a supply house. You go through the channels and you call that person in the supply house and he might be able to put you in touch with somebody in a salon. You've networked your way into a job possibility.

◎ I advise just calling up a salon—if you like the looks of it—and asking if you could come in to talk. Even if there is not a job at present, it certainly won't hurt for them to know you. Most people on the other end understand that this is the way the world works and will be inclined to cooperate.

◎ Every now and then, your networking overtures may lead to a door slamming in your face. If so, learn from it. There are people in the world who simply aren't very nice or very helpful or very sympathetic. Don't turn the behavior of these people into a personal rejection.

◎ When you visit a salon that you are considering as a possibility for prospective employment, bring along a checklist of items to help your reach a judgment. Is the receptionist friendly and warm, or rude and aloof? Are waste receptacles overflowing? How are people who work in the salon dressed? Are they wearing a uniform? If so, do you like the looks of it and would you feel comfortable wearing one? Compile a list of criteria and then, as you go from one establishment to the other, keep a record of your reactions.

- A sincere "Thank you" counts for a great deal. If anyone has helped you by answering questions over the telephone or by meeting with you, make sure you follow up their acts of kindness with your own. A brief note of thanks will stamp you in that person's memory as someone who knows how to do the right thing.

- When you call a salon to make an appointment for an interview, you may be told they are not hiring at this time. If you're lucky, they may offer to schedule an interview with you anyway. Under no circumstances should you regard this as a waste of time. To become skilled at interviewing, you need a lot of practice, so seize every opportunity. What's more, maybe they'll have a look at you and think you're just right for that other job that hadn't crossed their minds!

The All-Important Interview

The résumé and the networking are designed to get your foot in the door. So now that you've got that foot in the door, what's your next step?

- Even if you've learned about job-hunting protocol in beauty school or somewhere else along the way, it still seems like a good idea to start at the beginning. So when you're going for an interview, make sure, first and foremost, that you have identification with you. That means a Social Security number, a driver's license, the names and addresses of former employers, and the name and telephone number of the nearest relative not living with you. Don't leave home without these!

- First impressions count for a lot. That's just the way the world works. Think of how you've felt on occasions when a blind date comes to your door. Well, when you go into an interview, you're the blind date. That means your grooming and your wardrobe have to be impeccable. An interview is not the time for a halter top, no matter how hot the weather is, or jeans, or sandals, or T-shirts, or anything of the sort.

- Everything you wear has to be spotless and pressed. You are, after all, in the image industry. Your shoes have to be clean and in good repair. Keep your jewelry to a minimum. (No clinky-clanky jangle bracelets, please). And what about your hairstyle while we're at it? Is it fashionable and does it suit your face and features? If you aren't sure, ask someone who can tell you.

- I'll let you in on a secret: some people *hate* perfume. So why risk it? Leave it home that day.

- Carry a handbag or a briefcase, never both. You don't want to look like you're moving in on the poor guy.

Need a Wardrobe?

Many women find it difficult, if not impossible, to afford the two or three outfits necessary to project a confident and professional image when going out into the workplace. Fortunately, there are some wonderful nonprofit organizations that have been formed to address this need. These organizations receive donations of clean and beautiful outfits from individuals and manufacturers; these are then passed along to the women who need them. For more information, check out these two Web sites:

Wardrobe for Opportunity at www.wardrobe.org

Dress for Success at www.dressforsuccess.org

◎ Bring an extra copy of your résumé to the interview. Even if you've already sent one, the interviewer may not have it at his fingertips, so why be caught short?

◎ Anticipate questions. Obviously, you know that certain ones are going to be coming up. "Why did you leave your last job?" "Why do you want to work here?" You need to do your homework and make sure you've got some good responses handy.

◎ I tell the stylists I mentor to compile as many possible interview questions as they think they might encounter. Are you a team player? Are you flexible? What are your career goals? Are there any obstacles that would keep you from fulfilling your commitments? How would you handle a problem client? Who has influenced you most? How do you feel about retailing? Any and all of these may come up, so it helps to be ready.

◎ Role-playing your interview with friends or family can be very useful. Just make sure you're doing it with someone who knows how to be a serious critic.

◎ Some salons want you to demonstrate a service as part of the interview. They require an applicant to bring along a model and perform a cut and style. Check to see if this is a requirement and if it is, prepare for it.

◎ Punctuality is the number one rule. Never, ever, be late for an interview. Assume that if you're late, even by one minute, you've lost that job.

◎ To make sure you don't show up late for an interview, I advise scouting out the location a day in advance. Even if it's an hour away, make the trip and check the address. Go right up to the door so that you're not wandering around the next day, in a sweat, in some office park two minutes before you're due for the actual interview.

- Smile. When you walk in the door, when you leave, and whenever you can in between. A good smile is one of the best tools in your toolshed.

- Never lean on or touch an interviewer's desk or place your things on the desk. Some people are very territorial about their desks and you might get marks against you for this.

- Don't walk into an interview with a cup of coffee or a can of soda or food. And don't smoke or chew gum on an interview. Puh-leese!

- Sit up straight and speak clearly, just like your mother used to tell you.

- Whatever you do, do not criticize your past employers. An interview is not an occasion for you to air gripes. You'll only come off sounding like a malcontent or a loose canon.

- Always shake the hand of your interviewer at the end and say thank you for her time.

- There will come a critical point in the interview when the interviewer will sit back and say, "Now do you have any questions for me?" This is not a time to sit there looking pretty and shaking your head no. This is a time for you to seem like an intelligent, engaged person. Come prepared with a few questions. Not a whole barrage of them, just a few well-chosen ones. You might say, for instance, "Is there a job description and may I review it?" Or "Is there a salon manual?" Maybe you want to ask what kind of opportunities there are for continuing education or if there is room for advancement. It's your call, but just be sure to have some good questions handy when the time comes.

◎ Don't forget to follow-up your interview with a thank-you note. It's required. And it will give you the opportunity to restate your eagerness to fill the position, which could wind up being a key factor if the interviewer is choosing between two or three people.

◎ Keep in mind that there are certain questions that an interviewer does not have the right to ask and that you do not have to answer. Anything having to do with your race, religion, national origin or citizenship, age, marital status, sexual preference, disabilities, and physical traits. These are all off-limits. If one of these questions comes up, you should politely but firmly state that you do not think the question is relevant to the position being filled, and that you would like to focus on those qualities and attributes that are relevant. The message should sink in and your interviewer may actually wind up being impressed with your presence of mind.

Salary Negotiations

For some people, talking about money is painful. It doesn't have to be. Here are some good tips on negotiating around money.

◉ Do your homework. Know what the going rate is in the neighborhood for the position being filled. The more information you have, the more powerful your negotiating position will be.

◉ Negotiating for a job is not like negotiating for a car. If the negotiations work out, you and the person you're negotiating with are going to be living with each other, so operate out of good will. Don't assume an adversarial position. Also, it helps to realize that if you're being of-fered the position, that means that the firm you're negotiating with has made up its mind that you're the one for the job and so you both have the same goal: to make this happen.

◉ Know your priorities. If security is what races your motor, you may want more on the salary end and less on the commission. If you're an entrepreneurial type of personality, you may want the reverse.

◉ There are a lot of "extras" that may factor into your total package. Be aware of what they are. It could be vacation time, continuing education, flex time, or a six-month review with performance increases. Look into all of these and whatever else you can creatively come to, and keep them in mind when you're making your deal.

◉ Never lie. Don't say you made more than you did on your last job. On the other hand, you don't have to show all your cards. In a way, a salary negotiation is a little like a game of poker: a bit of bluffing, the old poker face. Maybe your first time out doing it, it will not go so well. But with practice, you may wind up winning a few hands.

◉ Make "fairness" the operative word in the negotiations. If cost of living has gone up, then it is only fair that your wages should rise accordingly. If your employer has budgetary restraints due to a slow economy, it is only fair that you take that into account.

◉ Bargaining is expected, but there comes a time when you run the risk of overkill. When you feel the offer is in the zone, then back off. Don't hold on for every last penny. Even if your demands are met, your employer may walk away from the experience feeling that he has hired a prima donna. Remember that negotiation is about give-and-take all around.

Chapter 12

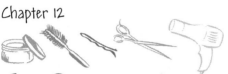

THE POSSIBLE DREAM

To some extent or another, most of us buy into the American dream. Owning your own house and having a nice car and money in the bank are fundamentals of the dream, and for those who have an entrepreneurial orientation, owning your own business completes the picture. The lure of owning one's own business is particularly strong in the cosmetology field where opportunities are so exciting. But keep in mind that starting your own business, or even working for yourself on a more limited basis, is an enormous responsibility. This chapter does not pretend to be your "starter kit" for growing a business, but it is full of the seeds of good ideas that you may choose to put into use at some future point.

Booth Rental

For anyone who wants to experience the rush of entrepreneurship without the full menu of headaches and stresses that can come with owning your own business, a booth rental (also known as chair rental) could be a good solution.

◎ I think booth rentals are just great. A booth rental allows you to become your own boss for very little money. Basically, your start-up expenses are your supplies and your rent. The rest is all profit with very little headache.

◎ Booth rentals work out well for many people, but you've got to realize that even though it's a pretty small and self-contained kind of business, it's still your business and nobody else's. That means that no matter how small it is, you've got all the worries about keeping the cash flow going. When you work for somebody else, you might have to worry about how good their cash flow is, but the expectation is that you will get your paycheck at the end of the week. Not so with booth rentals.

◎ Some people regard a booth rental is a nice "little" operation. Believe me, it's not so little. You've still got to be out there, getting and keeping the clients. And when you're up against the big chains, who are advertising and giving stuff away, that can be tough.

- Booth renting is great for someone who wants to work part time or is supplementing another income. Just make sure, before you get into it, that you have a large enough clientele to cover your costs.

- Unfortunately, I've seen people go into booth renting who thought they didn't have to go through all the hassle of owning your own business. Boy, were they in for a rude awakening. Booth renters have to keep scrupulous records for income tax and legal reasons, just like the big guys do. A booth renter has to carry malpractice insurance, which can be prohibitive, just like the big guys do. And there are still plenty of expenses connected to inventory, purchasing, and advertising. I'm not knocking it. You just have to know what you're getting into.

- This may be so basic as to sound almost stupid, but anyone going into booth renting has to remember a few critical things, like no one is paying you for vacations and if you're not there to do the work, you don't get the money. It's a whole other world.

- You've got to do the right thing by the IRS who will regard you as an "independent contractor." There are a lot of horror stories out there about getting caught by the IRS, but 99 percent of those stories really have to do with not following instructions or acting like the money you're making is play money. Establish a relationship with a reliable accountant right at the beginning of your enterprise to head off any problems at the pass.

- There are a lot of open-ended questions around booth-renting for both the renter and the landlord. For instance, who sets the prices? Are contracts or leases necessary? Do you have to have your own phone if you're a booth renter? The answers to these can be found by networking with people who have already taken the plunge and by looking at some of the literature out there on becoming a booth renter.

- In terms of booth rentals, the IRS is looking to see who has control over what. To protect yourself if you're audited, you have to show a contract to start out with. A lot of booth renters I know don't even have a contract, which is pretty crazy.

- Another thing the IRS looks for is to see if you're a booth renter who gets paid a commission instead of paying the landlord a flat rate. The IRS wants to see that booth renters collect their own money for services rendered.

- Another definition of a booth renter, from an IRS point of view, is whether you can come and go as you wish. If you're punching somebody's time clock, you're no booth renter.

- The IRS is also going to look to see how your scheduling is handled. You need to book your own services to establish that there is a clear separation between you—as booth renter—and the salon from which you rent. It's okay for you to use the salon's towels or shampoo, let's say, but you need to have your own telephone to show that you're separate. If you use the services of the salon's receptionist, that needs to be explained and written out in your agreement with the salon.

- In terms of a contract with the salon, you will, of course, want to consult an attorney, but among the guidelines to keep in mind is a minimum term, like six months, a 30-day clause for any contract changes, and a specification of liability issues. In terms of the latter, make sure to have your own insurance policy, including professional and liability coverage. This should probably cost you somewhere in the neighborhood of $300 a year.

- Even as a booth renter, you might want to incorporate. This helps protect your assets against any lawsuits and gives you certain tax benefits. Check with your attorney. Generally, fees to incorporate will run you about $1,000, but it could be well worth it. To incorporate, you need an Employer Identification Number (EIN) which you can get from the IRS or your local Social Security Administration office.

◉ Keep in mind that when you're a booth renter, you'll have to pay estimated quarterly taxes. Check with your accountant.

◉ If you're going to be retailing as a booth renter, which you will want to do to increase your revenues, remember that you will need a sales tax identification number. You can get this from your state sales tax agency for little money.

◉ If you're unclear about whether you're a booth renter or an employee of the salon, no matter what the paperwork says, ask yourself the following questions: Has the salon owner given you a key? Do you have your own telephone number? Do you schedule your own appointments? If the answer to these are "No," then you're not a booth renter.

Opening Your Own Salon

For some cosmetologists, opening their own salon is truly the pinnacle of their life experience. Certainly, such a step is a great accomplishment as well as a great responsibility. Owning your own business is a complex and sometimes very scary undertaking. Just the issue of having other people working for you can easily become one of the most difficult challenges you'll ever encounter. But it can also be exhilarating and, of course, extremely lucrative. Libraries and bookstores are filled with volumes about starting businesses, and you will have to do a great deal of reading and research to make sure you're going about it the right way if this, in fact, is your decision. But in this section, we will try to give you a brief overview of the process with tips from your fellow cosmetologists who have gone down that path.

"Location, Location, Location"

That's the famous saying when it comes to buying a house for the purposes of investment, but it holds every bit as true for buying a business.

- One of the world's worst ideas is a stand-alone salon. Even if it's gorgeous and fresh and new-looking, it will still have to overcome the hurdle of getting people to come to it when they could just as well go to another salon down the road that's next door to other shops that clients regularly use. Being able to kill two or three birds with one stone that way is, in the long run, going to prove a lot more attractive to the client than whether or not you've got terrazzo marble in the waiting area.

- In the world of residential real estate, there's a rule that says, "Be the best house on your block." Not so with the world of commercial real estate. You want to make sure you've got a good interface with your neighbors. If you're looking for a clientele that has style, taste, and affluence, don't surround yourself with dollar stores.

- If you're looking into a high-volume operation, you've got to check not only for street traffic but also you'll need to make sure that you're near some kind of public transportation.

- You've got to do the legwork. Become a private eye. Spend time in the neighborhood. Talk to business owners. You don't have to show your hand, but you can have pleasant, low-key, exploratory conversations with the person who owns the coffee house, the clothing store, the stationary store. You'll want to get an idea of the size, average income, and buying patterns of the local patrons. Do a lot of people go off to Florida for the winter? Is it an aging population? Is there a particular influx of a certain ethnic group? Some people, when they're thinking about starting a new business, actually do a stakeout, sitting in a car, let's say, for days, with a counter, figuring out how many people walk by on any given hour.

- Location is very important, but you could have a great location and if you hide your light under a bushel, what difference does it make? I've known owners who have put up the most discreet and subtle little signs. Hello? W⌄ the secret? And then there was this woma⌄ whose name was Szofia, the Hungarian spelling of Sophia. She named her shop Szofia's, which was charming and ethnic and all, but how many people do you think were able to get her number out of information or find her in the directory?

- Get a good look at the parking facilities. Parking can make or break a business. On a bad weather day, if you don't have convenient parking facilities, forget about it. And make sure you keep your parking lot well lit. Very important.

- An important factor with regard to location is who are you competing with? Sure, competition is the American way, but do you really want to go head-to-head with a salon that's already established? There's got to be a better way.

Getting Started

Once you've staked out a location, then you can go about the task of trying to make it happen. Here are some the things you'll need to think about.

- Don't even dream of opening up your own business without a business plan. You won't get anyone to lend you a cent, and that ads and relatives, not just the bank. to see something on paper.

own business can be extremely even terrifying at times. You'll feel totally lost at points. It happens to the best of us. The business plan is your map, your blueprint, your compass to point you on your way and keep you on track.

◉ The business plan gives you the big picture: what kind of personnel you'll need to hire; the salaries and benefits you have to factor in; a price structure; and a sense of your expenses like equipment, supplies, repairs, advertising, and taxes. You'll also have a mission statement as part of it, and that will be your bible to go back to when you're feeling like you may have strayed from your purpose.

◉ There are a ton of resources around to help you write your business plan. You'll find a great many good books, and there is also some excellent computer software for writing a business plan.

◉ I always suggest that people go to their local small business alliance for support when they're starting out. Most counties have these organizations where people from businesses come in to lend their expertise and mentor other people who are starting out. A lot of these organizations are funded so that they can give you 15 or 20 free hours of a consultant's time that you can apply to writing your business plan, let's say, or maybe starting up some aspect of the technology you'll need.

◉ An ironclad rule when starting your own business is to make sure that you've got enough capital. There will be plenty of slow stretches along the way. You may be convinced that when you leave your current situation, your clients will go with you, but slow down a little. A lot of clients are disinclined to make changes and you may find yourself scrambling to make up for the clients who won't come with you. A cushion of capital can help protect you against that contingency or against some other unexpected setback like an equipment failure, let's say.

◉ The start-up stage of your business involves getting the necessary licenses from your local, state, and federal agencies. Make sure you contact your local authorities regarding business codes and building regulations. Sales tax, licenses, and employment compensation are covered by state laws. You'll go to the federal level for payment of Social Security, unemployment compensation, and cosmetics and luxury tax payments.

◉ One of your most important decisions at the outset of your venture will be to determine what type of ownership works best for you. You might choose to be a sole proprietor or opt for a shared partnership, or you might want to form a corporation. All of these types of ownerships have their pros and cons, and you will want to explore them through reading materials, talks with friends and family, and discussions with lawyers, accountants, and so on.

◎ Recognize that in economic downturns, the priorities of your clients may shift from pampering themselves to stress relief. Make the appropriate image and promotional changes.

Surviving the Slow Times

Sufficient capital can see you through lulls, but there are other measures you can take to alleviate the crunch of these difficult periods.

◎ In slow times, shift your focus from customer to staff and concentrate on team building.

◎ Ratchet up education for everyone in these slow times.

◎ Have stylists spend more "quality time" with each customer.

◎ Plan special events like a product demonstration, for instance, or a hair show at the salon.

◎ Push gift certificates. Gift baskets, particularly in attractive containers like hatboxes, go a long way.

◎ Push prebooking. If a client doesn't know her schedule, try to book her anyway with the understanding that you'll call to confirm.

Buying an Existing Salon

Some of you may be presented with the opportunity to purchase an existing salon. This could prove an excellent choice, but, as with any big decision, you have to look at all sides of the picture.

◉ I know some people who have made out like bandits buying an existing salon. In some cases, very little remodeling was required, and considering the "move-in" condition, the price was more than right. I know other people, however, who bought a salon, thinking that their clientele was going to go along with them, and that can be a huge tactical error. Fixtures can move from one owner to the next, but make no assumptions about clients.

◉ All I can say is *caveat emptor*: let the buyer beware. I was once burned royally on fixtures. Ouch!

◉ I wouldn't dream of buying fixtures without working out some kind of warranty arrangement.

◉ Blood is thicker than water, but even if you're buying from blood, don't be shy about drawing up a written agreement. When it comes to buying a salon or making major purchases such as fixtures or equipment, use an account and a lawyer to draw up a written purchase and sales agreement to head off any future misunderstanding between the parties (even if that's you and your Aunt Matilda). You'll also need a complete and signed statement of inventory, detailing the goods and fixtures, and relative values of each item.

- The operative phrase here is: *Be careful.* If, for instance, there's a transfer of a note or a mortgage or a lease, you'll want to have a check done to make sure that there's been no default in the payment of debts.

- Don't forget to factor into your agreement your use of the salon's name and reputation for a prescribed amount of time. You're not just buying fixtures and a building: you're buying the identity that has brought people to that business over the years, at least until you create your own identity. The same applies to the clientele and their habits regarding services and purchasing. You'll want to arrange for access to that information. It makes total sense for that to be part of the deal.

- Don't forget about the noncompete clause of your purchase agreement. You don't want the guy you're buying the salon from to open another one across the street from you.

For Your Protection

There is considerable liability in owning your own business. Keep these pointers in mind.

◉ If you own your own business but don't own the building you're in, you will, of course, need a lease. Make sure that your lease specifies what is yours and what is the landlord's (that is, which fixtures you are within your rights to remove if you move to another location). You'll also want the lease to state what the landlord is responsible for (typically such repairs as painting, plumbing, electrical installation, and the like).

◉ One important point to have in any lease you sign is an option from the landlord that allows you to assign the lease to another person. That way, if you need to bring in another owner to share the business, or to even take over the business, you're entitled.

◉ Don't ever cut corners on insurance. You'll need liability, fire, malpractice, and burglary insurance, and you must make sure that they never lapse. Obviously, you have to be protected from things like fire and burglaries, but you wouldn't believe the people out there who'll sue you at the drop of a hat over nothing.

◉ The surest way to open yourself up to liability is by allowing yourself to think you're some

dical expert. Newsflash: you're not!
to diagnose, treat, or cure any med-
tion. That's what doctors are for, so
t of physicians handy that you can
refer to when dealing with clients who are having medical issues.

◎ I'm always surprised when people don't seem that grounded in the laws around cosmetology and the sanitary codes. Even people who own businesses sometimes act like it's a bunch of red tape that they can't really be bothered with. Well, you'd better be bothered with it, because if you make a mistake in that area, you run the risk of being put out of business altogether.

◎ As a business owner, you need to be absolutely scrupulous when it comes to keeping accurate records on employees, their salaries, lengths of employments, and Social Security numbers. There's a lot of coming and going in this field, and you can't afford to ever lose track. If you have someone else attending to all that, at least check their work!

Good Business Practices

Location means a lot, and talent and reputation mean a lot. But the foundation of a good business lies in good business practice. You need to be familiar with the fundamentals of business.

◎ I say, begin with networking. Look around at other salons in your city, see who's doing something that you admire, and make it a point to meet the owner of that business. By now, networking is such a buzzword in the business world that everyone recognizes its importance. Even owners of established businesses make time for networking because they realize that it's basic good business practice. And networking will offer you a wealth of information for free. Join a local business group or a chamber of commerce right at the start of your venture, and stay with it.

◎ Don't underestimate your start-up money. That's crucial. Before you open your business, determine how much capital you'll need to run it for at least two years. A great many businesses collapse because they've underestimated their start-up needs and then a crisis comes along, like a major equipment failure, let's say, and they're caught short.

◎ All business owners, even the smallest ones, have to recognize that there are management issues that they, as owners, have to become skilled at dealing with. If you do not have the background in management, you'll need to do a lot of reading or take some courses to come up to speed.

◉ To me, the two most important words associated with good business practice are quality control. A client needs to know that he is getting the best products and the best servicing, and if you, as the owner, can't monitor that and ensure it, then something is very wrong.

◉ So many of us have worked in shops that are run by human beings and in shops that are run by, for lack of a better word, nonhumans. People who manage people cannot do so effectively if they operate from a place of greed and fear and manipulation. It is very good business practice indeed to recognize the importance of employees and managers working together with respect for each other. Achieving harmony in your organization will enable everyone to work to their fullest potential.

◉ Training and continuing education should be a cornerstone of your business, for you as well as for everyone who works for you.

◉ Competitive pricing is a major issue in the running of your own business. Check regularly to see what other salons in your area are charging, and take into account the nature of their clientele and their location. Don't lag behind on prices or you run the risk of taking on the shabby patina of a budget operation.

Raising Prices

This is a big issue in the field. For starters, should you notify clients in advance? Some argue no. Dry cleaners don't tell you in advance when their prices are going up. The supermarket doesn't announce in advance a hike in cottage cheese. Discussing increases in advance may create too much discussion. An alternative to not announcing an increase in advance is to offer multilevel pricing. That way, if a client has a problem with the increase, he can be channeled to a stylist who will perform the service at the old price or he can pay the old price this time and the new one the next time, if there is a next time. Special promotions can salve the pinch for some clients, or you might even throw in some delicious freebie like a smoothie with a spa service. Some salons raise their prices yearly to get clients accustomed to the event.

 Business Record-keeping

Many a business has been broken on the wheel of poor record-keeping. If record-keeping does not seem like a skill that you will shine at, develop and put into place a system that will assure responsible record-keeping. Some of the following tips may sound basic, but there's no better place to begin than with the basics.

◎ Before you cut even one head of hair, line up an accountant or at least a bookkeeper. Most people don't have the interest or the aptitude to perform that kind of function by themselves, so don't feel you have to take on that area of work along with all your other duties. Your job will be to keep complete records to give to the accountant.

◎ Records are of value if they meet the "3 C's": they have to be *correct*, *concise*, and *complete*. They need to tell you what money has come in and what's gone out. In other words, income and expenses. Your income is what you make on services and retail sales. Your expenses include your rent, utilities, insurance, salaries, advertising, equipment, and repairs. You've got to hold on to every check stub, canceled checks, receipts, and invoices. Of course, your accountant will set up systems for you so you know just what to do.

◎ Some people tend to think that record-keeping is important mostly for when the IRS comes after you (if the IRS ever comes after you). What you need to realize is that all of your business transactions must be recorded in order for you to assess the value of the salon for prospective buyers, if that need should arise, or to arrange a bank loan or financing.

- You will have to keep certain financial records on a weekly or monthly basis so that you can make comparisons with other years. These records will indicate to you which services are doing well and which aren't. Daily records, on the other hand, give you the pulse of the business.

- Another important area of record-keeping has to do with the purchase of inventory and supplies. These records will hopefully keep you from buying too much or getting caught with buying too little of any one thing. They'll also clue you into pilfering—petty theft on the part of employees—which is a big problem in the field. A careful accounting of these inventory records will help you establish the net worth of your business at year's end.

Your Dream Salon

When you start a business from scratch or even, to a lesser extent, when you remodel an existing business that you've purchased, you will be faced with making some important design decisions. Here is some advice from those who have been there.

- When new owners talk about designing their salon, a lot of them start with the incidentals. "I want to have a granite reception desk" or "I want glass bricks setting off the consultation area." That kind of envisioning is fun to do, but you really have to remember to start with the basic principles that go into making a salon a viable space. These include easy access from the reception area to the floor, adequate aisle space and space for large equipment, a dispensary or back room, and plenty of storage space.

◎ Color is a crucial element in the salon. Your color scheme needs to be flattering to all and it should reflect the mood of the salon. Are you classic? Are you hip and trendy? Color yourself accordingly and consider consulting with a color expert so that you don't wind up painting the salon avocado green or something similarly uncomplimentary.

◎ Nothing is more important than good lighting. Go easy on the fluorescents and if you must use them, purchase quality bulbs that allow for good color representation in the hair color room. Good lighting is expensive, but you'll see that it translates into increased retail sales and you'll make your capital investment back in no time.

◎ Spacious changing rooms for the clients make a great impression. That cubby-in-the-locker-room feeling is a huge turnoff for some people.

◎ Pay close attention to the plumbing system you have installed. Who knows. You may want to put in a hydrotherapy tub one of these days and you don't want to be caught short with inadequate water pressure. The same holds true for your water heater. Don't purchase a puny one. You don't want to run out of hot water at any point in the day.

◎ You have to give careful consideration to all the codes concerning people with disabilities. You'll most probably need a special bathroom large enough to accommodate a wheelchair. I knew a person who created his own salon and didn't put in such a bathroom. When the time came to get a building permit and it became clear that the shop was not up to par in terms of handicap access, he had to make extensive renovations to correct the problem.

◎ People will talk to you about space and color and light, but the other crucial ingredient you have to work into your design plan is sound. One of the big attractions these days for clients coming to the salon is the experience of relaxation they can achieve while receiving services. Costs are an issue when it comes to soundproofing, but the good news is that it's not necessary to soundproof every wall. Just soundproof the quiet areas.

◎ Be aware of ventilation issues. As we all know, there are a lot of powerful chemicals being used in the salon.

Strictly Personnel

You may have the strongest showerheads and the plushest carpet and the best cappuccinos in town, but your salon is really only as good as the people who work there. That means that as an owner, you have to be able to hire and keep good staff. Let's have a look at some key areas of personnel.

Payroll and Employee Benefits

◎ To ensure a happy ship that is functioning to the height of its potential, the salon owner must be willing to share the success with the staff as it makes financial sense to do so. It's the right thing, and you can never go too far wrong doing the right thing.

◎ A powerful rule in business is to meet your payroll obligations before anything else. Some people try to pay off debts first, but that is morally not defensible.

◎ Pile on the benefits. It makes enormous fiscal sense in the long run because it helps to buy staff loyalty. And you will see that nothing is as valuable as staff loyalty.

◎ Don't even think about running a salon and dealing with personnel without having a firmly established structure of job reviews. It should be universally understood that raises come only with positive job reviews.

- Determine your policy around tipping and stick with it. Tipping is a real sticky-wicket in a lot of places, and can be more trouble than it's worth.

No Tipping?

Many salons have ruled out gratuities in the salon, feeling that tipping does not foster a professional image. Those salons that have abandoned gratuities have raised their prices to compensate for the average tipping income, believing that their prices reflect their worth and additional compensation is not necessary. Clients are freed up from the awkwardness of figuring out who and how much to tip, and there are never any challenges from the IRS because all income is declared. Salons who are now "tip-free" report that the hardest part of this change has been the planning and implementation, which must be done sensitively, patiently, and with understanding.

- If you're offering a commission system, put it in writing with a copy to each employee.

- Rules are for everyone. You can't make a non-smoking rule, for instance, but you get to do it in your office because you're The Owner.

- As an owner, you have to think of ways to instill motivation in your staff. Everybody gets stale after a while and motivation can weaken. I've found in our salon that a steady flow of incentives works wonders. We have prizes for lots of different things, and it keeps people on their toes.

Learn the Essentials of Management

Managing people is an art and a science, and hundreds of books have been written on the subject. Here is a "starter set" of tips for the budding manager.

◉ Honesty is key. Honesty is crucial. Honesty is what it's all about. Tell your people what you're thinking, when you're thinking it, whether it's positive or negative. Unless you're in the presence of a client, you'll want to provide honest feedback as close as you can to the event that you're inputting on.

◉ If you know anything about parenting—and after three kids, I can say I do—then you know about the power of positive reinforcement. This tool works just as well on the people who make up your staff. Everyone likes to hear good things said about themselves, so let people know when they've performed well. A regular diet of positive words acts as an invaluable cushion for those inevitable times when you have to give a staff member some negative feedback.

- Bring everyone into the loop. Don't let there be outsiders in the shop. When you have information regarding important salon decisions, pass it around.

- Think of management as a skill that you can teach to others. As an owner, you have had to work at your management skills and so are more evolved in that area than most of your workers are. But when you are making management decisions, it's a great idea to spend some extra time explaining to your staff what went into making those decisions. This way, they will develop more of a sense of that process, and may even evolve into management resources themselves.

The Salon Manual

The salon manual, also referred to as the operations manual, is a key tool in helping you establish a structure in the way you manage people. It should embody everything that you think is important and worthy about your business. When you buy a car, you get a manual that tells you where the latch is to open the hood, how to turn on the radio, and what to do if the "OIL" light goes on. Similarly, your salon operations manual should tell your employees where things are, how things work, and what to do in a full range of situations from how to handle

---

walk-ins to how to dispose of emery boards. The manual is your code that will help resolve disputes. As well, it should include your vision statement (where are you headed?) and your mission statement (how do you see going about realizing your vision?).

The Reception Area

One of the most critical members of your personnel team is your receptionist. The receptionist should operate in a reception area that is well conceived. The reception area needs to be stocked with business cards along with a prominently displayed price list that shows at a glance what clients should expect to pay for various services. Being a receptionist involves a variety of functions, from greeting clients to booking appointments to recommending services and retail items to the client, and consequently it demands a variety of skills. Here are some thoughts about what is needed up at the reception desk.

◎ You need to be a personality kid to be a really good receptionist. You can't sit there looking sullen or haughty. It's just not permissible. You need to greet clients by their names and to make them comfortable. You need to offer them a beverage if that's salon policy (as well it should be), and point to the basket of holiday cookies or candies or mini-muffins or whatever sweet little touch is there to brighten up the day. When announcing arrivals to the stylist, don't act like you're working in a railroad station. I always tell my receptionists that I never want to hear anything like "Gallagher. 12:30" coming from them. As busy as we may be, we will always have the time to say, "Mrs. Gallagher has arrived for her 12:30 appointment."

◉ The receptionist should think of himself as the host of a lovely party. In addition to making everyone comfortable, he should introduce people. "Mrs. Jones, I don't know if you've met Wanda, our nail technician." This is precisely what can lead to ticket upgrading.

◉ Receptionists have to look good. They don't need to be exquisitely gorgeous but they have to dress well, sit up straight, not wear excessive eye makeup or green hair, and they have to smile. A lot.

◉ Some receptionists develop a peculiar sense of ownership around the reception area and think that they can polish their nails there, have their salad on the desk, or do whatever they want. The answer is no.

◉ The receptionist has to have diplomatic skills. Often, she will be the one to take the heat from a disgruntled client. The receptionist cannot personalize this and should be skilled at dealing with such situations. This may take practice, so you, as salon owner, assuming you see potential in this employee, need to work with her to train for such situations.

◎ Work with your receptionist to create "scripts" for all different scenarios. The receptionist can embellish the script as he sees fit, but you want to provide a starting point.

◎ As a receptionist, you're going to act as a matchmaker. People may call you up cold and say, "I need to have my gray covered." The receptionist needs to know who in the salon is really good at that, or at styling extensions, or whatever.

◎ The receptionist should be highly knowledgeable about retail products. Giving the receptionist a bonus for sales is an incentive for her to become knowledgeable.

◎ The receptionist needs to understand that he is a member of a team. If there is significant down time up at the front desk, that's a great time for the receptionist to pitch in and straighten up something that needs straightening up or to fold some towels or do whatever to demonstrate a willingness to help.

Drumming Up Business

A final area of concern that a salon owner must address is that of promotion and marketing. You have a beautiful salon, a great staff, a good location, and competitive prices. So how do you get people to know about you?

◎ When I've taught classes to prospective salon owners, one of the first questions I always get is about advertising. I explain that advertising can be defined as any activity that promotes the salon in a good light. Not only newspaper ads and radio spots, but participating in a charity fashion show, for instance.

◎ No matter how big a budget you allot for advertising, there is no advertising in the world that can match the power of a satisfied client. This business is 98 percent about word-of-mouth and a happy client talking you up is worth more than a hundred newspaper ads.

◎ If you're looking for a general rule of thumb about advertising, the figure I've always heard is that your advertising budget should not exceed 3 percent of your gross income.

◎ Given the expense, if you're going to advertise, you have to make sure that every dollar you spend is used to the max. That means planning well in advance for holidays and special yearly events like proms, New Year's Eve, or June weddings.

◎ Newspaper ads may prove your most cost-effective way to advertise. Try a cut-out coupon in the ad so you can track how many new or returning clients the ad has attracted.

- Direct mail campaigns can be very effective but they can also be pricey. Consider using a good agency to create something for you. The piece should reflect the salon. In other words, if you're running a budget operation, it can look no-frills, maybe even a postcard, but it also has to be attractive, never cheap-looking. If you're aiming at the high end, you'll need high-quality stock on which to print the piece and the best quality graphics.

- The yellow pages is an important way to advertise. Make sure you have a listing, and you might even want to consider opting for one of the larger-size ads.

- Don't forget promotional items. Giveaway combs, emery boards, key chains, refrigerator magnets, calendars, and such are cheap to produce and turn up in all sorts of places that would otherwise be hard and expensive to target.

- If you've got a window, make the most of it. Be creative and informative, and highlight your retail products enticingly.

- Radio's nice, but it's more expensive than newspapers and harder to track.

- Forget about television unless you win the lottery.

- I've always relied to a large extent on community outreach. Ever since I started my salon, I'm everywhere: women's clubs, men's clubs, PTAs, church basements, radio, and TV talk shows. You ask me, you got me. I do my bit about style and presentation, which I have down to a fine turn, and I meet so many people. I volunteer at local bridal and fashion shows for just the same reason.

- Clients will refer others to you if they like you and particularly if you give them an added incentive to do so. I give any client who refers someone to me 10 percent off their next service or retail purchase.

INDEX